HUMAN-CENTERED LEADERSHIP IN HEALTHCARE

"Human-Centered Leadership in Healthcare: The Revolution Continues is a remarkable '2.0' treatise to the evolution of the authors' inspirational approach to leadership—connecting, awakening, upholding, and, of course, starting with self. As a longtime fan of relational leadership in all its forms, this book and its tenets speak deeply to me. It includes numerous practical and real-world examples, coupled with discussion and reflection questions in every chapter, providing a foundation for multiple learning experiences. This book will rekindle your belief that great human-centered leadership is not only possible, but also alive and well. Challenge yourself to use this approach to support both your own development and that of your teams. Happy reading!"

Rosanne Raso, DNP, RN, CENP, FAAN, FAONL
Editor-in-Chief, Nursing Management

"I am delighted to endorse *Human-Centered Leadership in Healthcare: The Revolution Continues.* This remarkable book builds on a powerful foundation to offer nurse leaders—and all healthcare professionals—a tested, evidence-based framework for leading with authenticity, courage, and compassion. The authors' collective voice weaves together deep scholarship and richly illustrative stories, guiding readers through the essential journey from self-awareness ("It starts with me") to fostering cultures of excellence, trust, and caring.

Whether you are a seasoned CNO, an emerging clinical leader, or a frontline nurse, *The Revolution Continues* will inspire and equip you to lead in a way that honors the shared human experience at the heart of healthcare. Read it, reflect on it, and watch as its principles transform your practice and your team."

Michelle Wallace, DNP, RN, TCRN, NEA-BC, FACHE
Chief Nursing Officer, Grady Memorial Hospital, Atlanta, GA

"Human-Centered Leadership in Healthcare: The Revolution Continues is a powerful and practical guide for transforming healthcare leadership from the inside out. Expanding on the original theory, the book introduces "Self" as a core dimension emphasizing well-being, reflection, and relational leadership as essential to sustaining teams and driving culture change. As today's workforce demands more meaningful connections, psychological safety, and purpose, this book offers timely solutions. It underscores the leader's critical role in shaping environments where people thrive, making it an essential resource for navigating the future of healthcare."

Renee Thompson, DNP, RN, FAAN, CSP
CEO & Founder, Healthy Workforce Institute®

"Human-Centered Leadership has been transformative for the nursing leaders—and leaders of nurses—across our organization. What makes it truly impactful is its ability to bridge theory and practice, offering practical, accessible strategies that bring human-centered leadership to life. With *The Revolution Continues*, this essential work deepens its relevance. A must-read for anyone committed to transforming healthcare through relational leadership and shaping the future of healthcare."

Brooke Baldwin, DNP, RN, CENP
SVP & Chief Nursing Executive, OHSU Healthcare
Associate Dean, Clinical Affairs, OHSU School of Nursing

"'It starts with you, but it's not about you.' What a powerful statement. Many times I have said that leadership is an inside job. Before we can answer the calling to serve others, we need to work on ourselves. When we got the inside right, the outside follows. Dr. Lucy Leclerc, Dr. Kay Kennedy, and Susan Campis have built a smart, researched-backed, and heartfelt book around this truth. The message I took away is that small, intentional human choices—made from a place of self-awareness and self-care—can ripple out and reshape an industry that's ready for change. It is time for healthcare leaders to move away from transactions and toward transformations and trust. This book helps show us the way."

Quint Studer
Co-Founder, Healthcare Plus Solutions Group and author of The Calling:
Why Healthcare Is So Special

"In *Human-Centered Leadership in Healthcare: The Revolution Continues*, the authors have crafted an essential guide that challenges traditional paradigms and inspires healthcare leaders to engage in a deeply transformative journey. This book is a call to action for leaders to prioritize human-centered approaches that make meaningful and lasting impacts on both patient care and organizational well-being.

With profound insights and evidence-based practices, this book builds upon its predecessor, guiding leaders to cultivate environments rooted in trust, resilience, and compassion. Through personal narratives, research-backed strategies, and practical tools, the authors illuminate the importance of starting from within—nurturing the Self—and extending outward to awaken, connect, and uphold our teams and colleagues.

Each chapter offers a rich tapestry of wisdom and actionable strategies, enabling leaders to navigate the complexities of modern healthcare with authenticity and courage. The book's focus on relational leadership fosters inclusion, collaboration, and empowerment, making this revolution not just a fleeting moment but a lasting movement toward excellence.

Human-Centered Leadership in Healthcare: The Revolution Continues is an indispensable resource that will inspire healthcare leaders at all levels to become architects of a future where human dignity thrives above rigid hierarchies. It challenges us to lead boldly, communicate with integrity, and build workplaces where we don't just work—we flourish together. Dive into this remarkable journey and discover how you, too, can be part of this revolution that champions the heart of healthcare leadership."

David Marshall, JD, DNP, RN, FAONL, FAAN
Senior Vice President & Chief Nursing Executive
Cedars-Sinai Medical Center
Los Angeles, CA

"Human-Centered Leadership in Healthcare: The Revolution Continues is more than a book—it is a bold and necessary manifesto for our time. In a healthcare environment that too often prioritizes metrics over meaning, this text returns us to the heart of what truly matters: human connection, relational leadership, and the well-being of those who lead and serve. The updated edition builds thoughtfully on the original framework, offering tested strategies, powerful narratives, and actionable insights that resonate deeply with the realities nurse leaders face today.

As a chief nurse executive, I see firsthand the urgent need for leadership that is courageous, compassionate, and grounded in purpose. This book delivers exactly that. From the integration of caring science to the crosswalks with national standards, it bridges the academic, operational, and human dimensions of leadership in a way that is both practical and profoundly transformational.

This is not just a guide for individual development—it is a call to collective action. Whether you are at the bedside, in the boardroom, or shaping the future of nursing education, *The Revolution Contin-*

ues equips you to lead with clarity, authenticity, and heart. I recommend it wholeheartedly to every nurse leader who believes that the future of healthcare must be built on human-centered values."

Anne Marie Watkins, DNP, MSHCA, RN, CENP
SVP/System Chief Nursing Executive and Assistant Dean of Nursing Education
University of California, Irvine Health

"*Human-Centered Leadership in Healthcare: The Revolution Continues* is a transformative guide that redefines what it means to lead with purpose, compassion, and authenticity in today's complex healthcare landscape. Grounded in research, previous work and application, and rich with lived experience, this book empowers nurse leaders to embrace their humanity, nurture their well-being, and ignite meaningful change—from the inside out. In today's challenging healthcare landscape, what could be more important? This is a must-have resource!!"

Tim Porter-O'Grady, DM, EdD, APRN, FAAN, FACCWS
Senior Partner, Health Systems, TPOG Associates, LLC. ATL/PHX
Clinical Professor, Emory University, NHWSN, Atlanta, GA
GCNS-P Wound Specialist (AZ, OH)

HUMAN-CENTERED LEADERSHIP IN HEALTHCARE

The Revolution Continues

It starts with you, but it's not about you!

LUCY LECLERC, KAY KENNEDY, AND SUSAN CAMPIS

American Nurses Association

uleadership

About the American Nurses Association

The American Nurses Association is the only full-service professional organization representing the interests of the nation's 5 million registered nurses through its constituent/state nurses associations and its organizational affiliates. ANA advances the nursing profession by fostering high standards of nursing practice, promoting the rights of nurses in the workplace, projecting a positive and realistic view of nursing, and by lobbying the Congress and regulatory agencies on healthcare issues affecting nurses and the public.

American Nurses Association
8403 Colesville Rd., Ste. 500,
Silver Spring, MD 20910

Library of Congress Control Number available upon request.

ISBN-13

Print	978-1-963052-37-4
ePDF	978-1-963052-38-1
ePUB	978-1-963052-39-8
SAN	851-3481

Notice

No responsibility is assumed by the publishers for any injury and/or damage to persons or property as a matter of products liability, negligence, or otherwise, or from any use or operation of any methods, products, instructions, or ideas contained in the material herein. Because of rapid advances in the medical sciences, in particular, independent verification of diagnoses and drug dosages should be made.

For all healthcare leaders.
Your every action, every moment,
fuels our collective movement.

Contents

Acknowledgments

Bringing this book to life has been a journey—one that started with a vision but continues to evolve with every conversation, collaboration, and insight from the nurse leaders shaping healthcare today. It hasn't been a solitary process; it has been built through shared experiences, challenges, and unwavering commitment to amplifying voices that drive change. Along the way, our partners in this adventure—Louis, John, and Mark—have offered steady support, patience, and countless moments of encouragement when we needed them most.

We are especially grateful to the global community of nurse leaders whose resolute commitment to Human-Centered Leadership in Healthcare® continues to inspire systemic transformation. Their dedication to fostering inclusive, compassionate, and psychologically safe healthcare environments pushes the profession forward in ways that ripple beyond hospital walls and into the lives of patients, families, and communities. Their collective wisdom, advocacy, and action have made this work possible, and we are honored to amplify their voices in these pages.

Finally, we want to give a big shoutout to the American Nurses Association publishing team for their creativity, encouragement, and steadfast support. Thank you for believing in us and in the power of this work to shape a more inclusive, human-centered future in healthcare.

Foreword

The new edition of Human-Centered Leadership in Healthcare is an evolved level of focused leadership for a new era in healthcare. Acknowledging leaders' humanity and self-care, first, becomes the caring science core of leadership. Human-Centered Leadership continues to be a revolution in contrast to dominant system-focused models of leadership, paving the way forward for true transformation from within. It is from this larger caring science consciousness of leadership where challenges become opportunities for creativity and solutions, which inspire, inform, and ignite new possibilities for all.

Your Human Caring Leadership continues as a beacon of hope and a guide for self and systems. The new edition will continue to serve as a solid touchstone for a healthcare system in dramatic need of change from within.

Jean Watson, PhD, RN, AHN-BC, FAAN, LL (AAN)
Founder/Director, Watson Caring Science Institute
Distinguished Professor/Dean Emerita, University of Colorado, Denver, CON
jean@watsoncaringscience.org
www.watsoncaringscience.org

Preface

Leadership in healthcare is not simply a title—it's a commitment, a calling, and, in many ways, a revolution. *Human-Centered Leadership in Healthcare: Evolution of a Revolution* marked the beginning of a shift—a call for nurse leaders to embrace leadership not just as a role, but as a deeply human-centered, relational practice. Now, with *Human-Centered Leadership in Healthcare: The Revolution Continues*, we build upon the foundation we laid, testing, validating, and evolving what we know to ensure that this movement is not fleeting, but lasting, persistent, and transformational.

This revolution did not begin in boardrooms or formal leadership seminars—it began with coffee, conversation, and candid reflection. We sat together, three nurse leaders with decades of experience, sharing stories that in equal parts were joy and challenge, fulfillment and exhaustion, impact and sacrifice. We recalled the leaders who inspired us, and those whose leadership left us feeling unseen. We talked about our own leadership—where we thrived, where we struggled, and how, too often, the demands of the job pushed self-care, self-awareness, and self-compassion to the sidelines. In those conversations, we realized that we were not alone in our experiences. And if we felt this way, countless other leaders did, too.

That realization propelled us forward. Week after week, coffee cup after coffee cup, we refined and tested the ideas that would form the foundation of Human-Centered Leadership in Healthcare®. What started as dialogue became a framework. And what began as theory was put into practice, examined in real-world settings, challenged, adapted, and strengthened. Leadership, after all, is not static. It's dynamic, evolving, and shaped by the people who engage in it every day.

This book is not a conclusion—it is a continuation. A testament to the consistent, deliberate work required to lead with authenticity, courage, and inclusivity. The revolution is not over. It is unfolding in every patient interaction, leadership decision, and system we choose to challenge and improve. It starts with you, but it's not about you. And together, we push forward.

A Few Words About This Book

Leadership is a reflection of the shared human experience, evolving alongside the challenges, relationships, and aspirations that shape healthcare. This book was born from real-world conversations, research, and lived experiences—a response to the persistent need for bold and passionate nurse leaders who embrace leadership as a human-centered profession. From the bedside to the boardroom, Human-Centered Leadership in Healthcare (HCL-HC) has emerged as more than a framework—it is a tested, validated, and evolving approach that challenges conventional paradigms of what "good" leadership looks like in today's complex, rapidly changing world. Guided by complexity and caring science, the timeliness of this updated text will illustrate that, indeed, a human-centered leadership approach in healthcare is an idea that's time has come.

In Part I, we present updated research studies, evidence-based projects, and global dissemination to illustrate the scope of the revolution of HCL-HC. Part II turns inward, guiding you through the most often neglected dimension of leadership: yourself. The big "aha" in Part II is the evolution of the theory to identify the *self* as a separate and unique dimension of HCL-HC. We share the mindset of "It starts with me" and the language of "I matter" associated with this dimension. Well-being, self-nurturing, self-compassion, self-awareness, and mindfulness are not luxuries—they are the foundation of resilient, sustainable leadership. The human-centered leader understands that well-being fuels impact, and only by nurturing oneself can a leader truly uplift and model for those around them.

In Part III, we explore the outward-facing dimensions of the human-centered leader—the Awakener, the Connector, and the Upholder—and bring these dimensions to life through exemplars, stories from the field, and the voices of research participants whose experiences translate theory into tangible practice. Finally, in Part IV, we provide an expanded library of actionable strategies to strengthen the attributes of human-centered leaders in their daily work. This section is designed to appeal to the most frequently requested ways to operationalize Human-Centered Leadership (HCL) through: *Human-Centered Communication*, *Human-Centered Design*, *Human-Centered Understanding*, and *Human-Centered Belonging*. These techniques are designed to develop the people who lead the people, ensuring that leadership is not just an individual journey but a collective movement. Part V renews the call to action as an "idea that's time is now" and one that is nearing the tipping point for monumental change in prioritizing relational leadership as the way forward. Finally, the Appendices are filled to the brim with updated information to guide leaders in practice and academia to build HCL-HC into actionable behaviors and outcomes.

This book is an invitation—an opportunity to step into the revolution of HCL-HC. Leadership is not static. It is persistent, evolving, and deeply personal. We believe that somewhere in these pages, you'll recognize yourself. And just maybe, you'll recognize the nurse leader you would follow to the ends of the earth.

Voice. A brief note about the voice used in this book. While there are clearly three authors, the manuscript is represented as the collective voice of one. Our research and the contents of this book are infused with the voice of nursing. You'll find instances when we share stories from a personal "I" perspective. These stories come from either our own experiences or have been garnered from experiences shared by colleagues over the past 30 plus years. Stories from this personal perspective are the greatest connectors, and we believe you'll find something familiar in many of them. Rest assured, names and minor details have been altered to ensure anonymity in both the positive and not-so-positive anecdotes. All scholarly or evidence-based information is cited to give credit to the appropriate author or source. We also used the collective "we" when aiming to share the united voice of the authors. The goal is to prevent you from wondering which one of the authors wrote this or that. Instead, we want you to visualize the writing as the voice of nursing.

Audience. The book is designed for a wide audience in nursing and healthcare. We envision utility in book clubs for practice settings, such as shared governance councils or the chief nursing officer's executive team. Practice settings could also use this book as a foundation for leadership programs, especially those on a journey to excellence. This updated book also includes a crosswalk of the *American Organization of Nurse Leader Core Competencies* (2022) with HCL-HC dimensions and attributes.

The alignment between leader competencies and the relational style of HCL could guide leadership curricula and development plans (Appendix I). We also see this text as a viable option for nursing programs from BSN to MSN to DNP. With mindful intention, we aligned the American Association of Colleges of Nursing (2021) *The Essentials: Core Competencies for Professional Nursing Education*'s Domain 10 on Personal, Professional, and Leadership Development with the evidence-based attributes of HCL-HC (Appendix G). We see this as an upstream effort to influence the leaders of tomorrow with a nursing-centric and human-centered way of leading. Finally, we created thought-provoking reflection prompts to be used in either practice or academia, as well as discussion questions for each chapter. The reflections are aimed at individuals while the discussion questions are designed for just that, igniting groups to talk, to innovate, and to consider alternative ways of being. These are the keys to activating the learning in each chapter. Each chapter also includes a list of cited references as well as recommended reading to further engage thought and expand the horizons of learning.

PART I

The Revolutionary Theory Evolves

The evolution of an idea includes an accumulation and integration of change over time. Human-Centered Leadership in Healthcare® (HCL-HC) was originally introduced as a constructivist reflection of modern healthcare leadership grounded in the idea that effective leaders in complex systems prioritize their own well-being. The leader is then equipped to turn their energy outward to Awaken, Connect, and Uphold their teams and colleagues. Through rigorous testing of the theory with real-world leaders and teams, HCL-HC has expanded into a more mature version with nuances related to mindset, language, measurement, and how to put it into action. Read on and discover the ongoing research that's informed the latest and greatest version of HCL-HC.

CHAPTER 1

On the Shoulders of Giants

If I have seen further, it is by standing on the shoulders of giants.

—Sir Isaac Newton, English scientist

Have you ever looked up at the night sky and felt an unexpected sense of connection—like you're part of something bigger? There's something about stargazing that reminds us we're not alone. Across time and cultures, people have looked up to the sky with curiosity, wonder, and even a hint of hope. The same stars that guided ancient travelers, inspired storytellers, and fueled scientific discoveries are still shining above us today. It's a reminder that no matter how much the world changes, we're all linked through the shared human experience.

And that brings us to Human-Centered Leadership in Healthcare (HCL-HC). Like the stars, leadership evolves, shaped by new ideas, shifting landscapes, and the needs of those it serves. What began as a concept grew into a theory, then into a guiding philosophy—one that embraces the complexity and unpredictability of modern healthcare while staying rooted in the values that have always mattered.

In this chapter, we'll explore how this approach took shape and why it continues to be a powerful force in nursing and healthcare leadership today. Come along as we trace the path of a theory that, much like the stars, has the potential to illuminate the way forward.

What If Copernicus Had Just Kept His Mouth Shut?

Robust theories continuously unfurl, emerge, and take shape to stand the test of time. Theories are inextricably connected to practice and practice to the dynamic emergence of theory. Just like when Copernicus first proposed that the Earth was a planet like Jupiter that circled the Sun. This was a revolutionary and unpopular idea that had to be tested because back then the more widely held belief was that the Earth was the center of the universe. Unfortunately, it was 1515 and there were no powerful telescopes to help him test the theory. By 1610, one of his contemporaries, Galileo, pointed his telescope to the night sky and saw that moons orbited Jupiter, and he documented the phases of Venus to prove that the planets do indeed orbit the Sun. Next, Kepler and other scientists built on Galileo's and Copernicus' theories, developing the mathematical equations still used today to predict the movement of planets. As time passed and history moved along, you might recall how an apple changed everything, and Isaac Newton added to Kepler's theory of planet movement by defining motion. From there, Newton shifted the scientific perspective to the Laws of Motion and Gravity. You're probably on the edge of your seat, wondering who gained an advantage over Newton. If you said Einstein, you get a gold star. In the early 1900s, Einstein honored Newton's ideas but added an element related to relativity. The Theory of Relativity didn't replace Newton's laws of motion and universal gravitation, which are still used today to launch satellites; rather, the Theory of Relativity was a more inclusive representation of Newton's theory. Were the theories of Copernicus, Galileo, Kepler, Newton, and Einstein inaccurate? No. Evidence supported each theory, generated accurate expectations, used a specific frame, and most importantly paved the way for new avenues of research, thinking, and practice. If Copernicus had kept his mouth shut, perhaps the journey to the scientific understanding of physics would have looked quite different. Thankfully, in today's highly technological world and in part due to the work of giants such as Copernicus and his colleagues, research and the evolution of theories don't take 400 years. If that were the case, we wouldn't have much to share about HCL-HC. What you're about to read is our own Copernicus story but one within a world that is much more connected than in the 1500s.

Which Came First, the Theory or the Practice?

A theory evolves when new questions are asked, new contexts emerge, and new frames are used to understand and explain the phenomenon. In a review of the evolution of nursing research, Stolley, Buckwalter, and Garand (2020) wrote that theories also evolve when new evidence is brought forward. Theories are not static, rather they can be compared to a living organism that matures, ages, changes, and adapts to an ever-changing world. Theories are also informed by perspectives and contexts. HCL-HC provides an exemplar of how a theory really does grow and change. Since the original constructivist grounded theory was published in 2021, we couldn't have imagined the groundswell of interest in this contemporary, relational, and healthcare-specific leadership theory. Nurses from around the globe identified with the shared mindset of leading from the perspective of a shared human experience. We discovered you can't just "drop the mic" and walk away. Nurse scientists, leaders, and academics were eager to test the theory. And we were delighted to partner with them. HCL-HC looks a lot like its original self of four years ago, but real-world application with nurses and teams has cultivated growth with roots and branches. The theory is not bigger, but it's definitely better. It's better because science challenged the theory (and us) with hard questions such as "What does it look like in practice?", "Does it make a difference in outcomes, for nurses and patients?", "How do you measure it?", and "How do we integrate the theory into graduate education?".

These questions and many others guided the evolution and related work over the past four years. HCL-HC was first introduced as a contemporary theory, and to some, a movement, grounded in the concepts of complexity. The original theory focused on leadership from the "inside out." As we journeyed across the United States and worked via the virtual world with global colleagues, the theory evolved in front of our eyes. As nurse leaders from practice and academia tested the theory by putting it into action, some significant advances reminiscent of Newton's apple drop developed. Here are some of the highlights:

- **"Self"** evolved as a distinct dimension, which expanded the theory from the previous three dimensions of Awakener, Connector, and Upholder.
- **A validated instrument** was developed to measure the four dimensions of HCL-HC from different perspectives: Self-Assessment, Others (Direct Reports), and Colleagues.

- A **mindset** and **language** capturing the essence of each of the four dimensions emerged.
- A transformative roadmap was crafted to help leaders evolve personally and professionally, bringing the four dimensions to life in an actionable way: **Being, Knowing,** and **Doing.**
- A connecting theme of **relational leadership** surfaced: relationship with Self, first, and then the outward focus on relationships with others.
- As appetite and demand for HCL-HC grew, we developed a **Certified Facilitator Course** in which participants are equipped with the knowledge, skills, and tools to effectively teach and promote these leadership principles. The course combines theoretical frameworks with practical application, enabling facilitators to foster relational and HCL practices within their organizations.

So, to answer the initial question in this section, "Which came first, the theory or the practice?", I would challenge you to answer right now to yourself. Do you think human-centered leaders existed before we did our original research in 2020? We believe the answer is yes. The practice was there, but it had not been named. In this instance, we believe the practice came before the theory, but practice is now informing and refining the theory.

The Intent and Context

In our 2021 introduction to HCL-HC, we used the metaphor of a hospital's physical architecture to highlight the importance of the human aspect of healthcare (Kennedy, Leclerc, & Campis, 2021). Just as the steel beams and concrete foundation of a hospital become invisible yet essential supports, the human architecture—nurses, doctors, and the entire team—provides vital care. Registered nurses, who form the largest part of the healthcare workforce, are like the invisible beams, working tirelessly round-the-clock 365 days a year. Expanding this metaphor beyond a single hospital to city-wide and national levels, nurses remain the backbone of healthcare. With nearly 4.7 million nurses in the United States, they are the invisible architecture that ensures continuous care (National Council of State Boards of Nursing, 2024). Just as the physical structure of a hospital supports its purpose, nurses support the humans entrusted to their care, maintaining the health and well-being of patients every minute of every day.

The intention of this book is to update the original introduction of HCL-HC with real-world examples of the theory in action. We will also share real-world research done by not just us, but others from around the world who are integrating HCL into practice environments. As we consider this strong sense of purpose and commitment to care for others, the HCL-HC approach will assist you in putting a name to the qualities and attributes of the leader you may already be and the leader you aspire to be. The primary tenets of HCL-HC will help you identify how effective leaders start with self and then organically emanate their influential energy outward to their teams and their patients. In this book, we will walk you through a series of steps to identify and recognize HCL-HC attributes that already exist within your leadership style and will challenge you to consider how to strengthen other HCL-HC attributes that might not be as evident to you. You will be challenged to do a good bit of self-reflection and self-examination because, as we say in HCL, "It starts with you, but it's not about you."

Why does HCL-HC zero in on healthcare leaders and, specifically, nurse leaders? Remember, nurse leaders are those leaders at the point of service from the bedside to the boardroom and all roles in between. To answer the question, HCL-HC did not originally intend to "target" a certain population; rather, the theory and approach continue to emerge through ongoing research and construction of meaning. This means we've collaborated with nurses and interprofessional teams around the world to validate the dimensions, expand the theory, measure the dimensions, validate how the dimensions are operationalized in practice, and explore connections between HCL-HC

INTENTIONS

- Discover how the theory has been updated to reflect real-world practices.
- Dive into the research that supports the updated theory and associated outcomes.
- Identify ways you can put HCL-HC into practice, just like the many nurses and leaders who've paved the way over the past few years. Their stories will inspire you!
- Learn about strategies to align dimensions of the human-centered leader at all levels of nursing education (BSN, MSN, and DNP) by focusing on alignment with the ANA *Code of Ethics for Nurses* (2025) and AACN *Essentials* (2021). See Appendices D and F.

and outcomes. Because evidence is the foundation of practice, in the following chapter, we'll describe the various studies we've had the honor to do with experts across the globe. The primary intentions of this book are to share with you the new and improved theory, the research behind it, and the exciting outcomes-based ways it's been put into practice. Our hope remains the same, that you'll feel as if you're connecting with an old friend, that leader you knew years ago when you were a new nurse, or that leader you now work alongside. We also hope you'll recognize yourself.

Discussion Questions for Groups

By addressing the following questions in a discussion with colleagues, we can better understand the potential for nursing to evolve beyond traditional methods and embrace a contemporary, relational leadership style that aligns with the ongoing changes in society (Appenidx J).

1. Movements often undergo phases of growth, resistance, and adaptation. How do you see this pattern in the context of nursing leadership today?
   - Do you believe the profession is currently experiencing a phase of resistance to change, or is it more adaptive and open to new ideas?
   - What indicators would suggest that nursing is ready for a paradigm shift in moving from traditional or transformational leadership to HCL-HC?
2. Consider the role of grassroots activism in the evolution of social movements. How can grassroots efforts within nursing contribute to a broader transformation in the field related to leading in a relational way?
   - What are some examples of grassroots initiatives that have successfully brought about change, and how can these principles be applied to nursing?
   - How important is it for nurses to engage in advocacy and activism to promote a new vision for the profession's future?
3. Finally, discuss the importance of intergenerational collaboration in the evolution of movements.
   - How can newer generations of nurses learn from the experiences and lessons of those who came before them, and vice versa?
   - In what ways can this collaboration drive innovative approaches and solutions in nursing leadership and practice?

Reflection Questions for Individuals

As you consider the fact that change is inevitable within your own life, profession, and organization, how can you develop a mindset to better manage and even welcome new ways of thinking and leading? What's one small thing you could do differently that would influence how you view change? Consider how evidence and research could play a role.

____

____

____

____

____

References

American Association of Colleges of Nursing. (2021). *The essentials: Core competencies for professional nursing education.* Retrieved from https://www.aacnnursing.org/Portals/0/PDFs/Publications/Essentials-2021.pdf

Kennedy, K., Leclerc, L., & Campis, C. (2021). *Human-centered leadership in healthcare: Evolution of a revolution.* Morgan James.

National Council of State Boards of Nursing. (2024). *Active RN licenses.* Retrieved from https://www.ncsbn.org/nursing-regulation/national-nursing-database/licensure-statistics/active-rn-licenses.page

Stolley, J. M., Buckwalter, K. C., & Garand, L. (2000). The evolution of nursing research. *Journal of the Neuromusculoskeletal System JNMS: A Journal of the American Chiropractic Association, Inc, 8*(1), 10–15.

Recommended Reading

Arnone, J. M., & Fitzsimons, V. (2015). Plato, Nightingale, and Nursing: Can you hear me now? *International Journal of Nursing Knowledge, 26*(4), 156–162. doi: 10.1111/2047-3095.12059

Ballard, N., Tussing, T., & Wei, H. (2022). Developing effective leadership skills and capacity. In H. Wei & S. Horton-Deutsch (Eds.), *Visionary leadership in healthcare: Excellence in practice, policy, and ethics* (pp. 87–115). Sigma Theta Tau International.

CHAPTER 2

Proof in Practice

Facts are stubborn things; and whatever may be our wishes, our inclinations, or the dictates of our passions, they cannot alter the state of facts and evidence.

—John Adams, American Founding Father and Second President of the United States

The words of John Adams, "Facts are stubborn things," really helped define our intention over the past few years to explore the "so what?" question of Human-Centered Leadership in Healthcare (HCL-HC). Because a theory is just that, a theory, and research is filled with hypotheses or "what ifs," we stepped into the river of inquiry not knowing if this would be a bust or a boom. Thankfully, we found it to be the latter, but you can form your own opinion as you continue to read. To make the connection between clinical practice and leadership practice, let's go through a clinical example of how evidence informs practice and vice versa. As you know, in healthcare, we rely on "best practices" and demand evidence to support the care of patients and our communities. We expect a patient who arrives in the emergency department with symptoms of a stroke to receive care that reflects decades of evidence. From the moment the patient arrives, the clock starts, and a series of time-sensitive actions by providers and nurses is initiated. This includes brain imaging, IV access, STAT labs, NIHSS exams, 12-lead ECGs, oxygen saturation and vital signs monitoring, and the administration of tPA Alteplase—all within the emergency department. The evidence-based care continues throughout the patient's stay and long after discharge to home or rehabilitation. In fact, the evidence used in that stroke patient's care lasts a lifetime. According to the American Heart Association's recent guidelines, when evidence-based practices are utilized by healthcare teams, patients are more likely to survive and avoid readmission within the subsequent 30 days (Ashcraft et al., 2021). Think about that. Receiving specialized and evidence-based care provided by skilled human resources increases the likelihood that stroke patients will not only survive the initial episode but also recover successfully. This is an example of connecting evidence to outcomes, and in a theoretical sense, we're connecting a set of ideas and concepts to measurable results.

What if we looked at leadership in a similar way? Which leadership approach do you subscribe to? Is it based on evidence? Is it specific to healthcare? Has anyone proven that it improves measurable outcomes, such as a healthy work environment, patient satisfaction, staff retention, reduced errors, or improved just culture? No need to answer right now. You'll have plenty of opportunities to consider these questions as we navigate the evolving theory of HCL-HC and the research that illustrates the connection to outcomes.

HCL-HC is a theory that's maturing due to the research and evidence-based projects completed in recent years. The real-world application of this contemporary, relational style has been shown to contribute to cultural transformation within hospitals and healthcare organizations. What follows is an overview of the research and evidence-based inquiry we performed over several years to refine, develop, and redefine the qualities of the leaders we would follow to the ends of the earth. What's even better and more beautiful is that we're not the only ones doing the research! External, third-party validation of HCL-HC will show you the evidence from a new perspective.

Join us as we delve into the realms of theory and research. Keep in mind that those stroke protocols that save lives and improve care started with theories and research.

Charting the Course of Inquiry

Self: If it had been a snake, it would have bitten us!

As we started working with nurse leaders to coach and mentor on how HCL-HC could be implemented into practice, we consistently heard from them that our model and theory were missing something. Have you ever been so immersed in an activity that you missed the most important part? Consider a musician so focused on perfecting a difficult section of a song that they miss the audience's positive reactions during the rest of the performance. Or a hiker so absorbed in reaching the summit that they fail to appreciate the stunning views along the trail. We experienced this through the process of calling out and naming the dimensions of HCL-HC. While we originally identified the essence of HCL-HC through the constructivist grounded theory research process with the tagline, "It starts with you, but it's not about you," we failed to name Self as a distinct dimension. The published research in 2021 identified three dimensions: Awakener, Connector, and Upholder (Leclerc, Kennedy & Campis, 2021; Kennedy, Leclerc, & Campis, 2021). Where in the world was Self?! We were too busy hiking the proverbial research trail that we missed the stunning view that would be named "Self." Self was right there in front of us, yet we had not called it out. As the idiom goes, "If it had been a snake, it would have bitten us!" This is a real-world example of how practice informs theory. Tuck that away for your next graduate theory class. Revising the theory and model to specifically add the dimension of Self is one of the most significant updates over the past few years. Remember Galileo? We pointed our newly discovered "telescope" to the real-world nurses we worked with in the early years of 2021 to 2022, and there it was. Just like Galileo discovering that the planets orbited the Sun, we realized that the outward-facing dimensions of the Awakener, Connector, and Upholder were orbiting the most primal and important dimension of the Self.

The journey to identifying Self began as we spent 2021, during the height of the pandemic, working with a rural hospital in Louisiana. Over a nine-month on-site implementation of HCL-HC, working side-by-side with an interprofessional leadership team that included the CEO and CNO, the focus on American Association of Critical Care Nurses Healthy Work Environment standards as a measure of potential influence opened our eyes to the absolute necessity of prioritizing Self (Leclerc, Strenge-McNabb, Thibodeaux, Campis, & Kennedy, 2022). If you read Leclerc et al.'s (2022) publication, you'll notice that Self is not called out as a separate dimension; however, the team included strategies related to Self in the implementation at that rural hospital. The implementation included leader mentoring in HCL-HC, structured action plans with individual leaders based on American Association of Critical Care Nurses Healthy Work Environment surveys, live on-site or virtual learning labs every two weeks for a total of 18 one-hour interactions (Shared Leadership, Professional Development Plans, Mindfulness, Self-Awareness, Self-Compassion, Resilience, etc.), and a web-based HCL-HC program with six levels of "Learn-Do-Inspire" microlearning activities designed to activate engagement within the learning community (Leclerc et al., 2022). The concept of Self was integrated into the curriculum through two avenues while not being called out as a separate dimension: (1) the web-based program had an entire module dedicated to "It starts with you . . ."; (2) the on-site and virtual learning labs balanced outward-facing strategies with Self strategies such as Self-Awareness and Self-Compassion. It would take time and additional, secondary examination of the "It starts with you . . ." content and field observations from additional healthcare settings to formally define what Self means in the context of HCL-HC. It wasn't until a January 2023 publication by Leclerc and Pabico that Self was formally published as a distinct dimension (Leclerc & Pabico, 2023).

From there, we refined the HCL-HC curriculum by deepening our focus on the dimension of Self and moving to virtual, real-time sessions. Trading prerecorded content for live interaction was like stepping out of a photograph and into a conversation. It transformed the experience from a static snapshot into a living, breathing exchange—where empathy, presence, and connection could unfold in real time. After all, you can't teach about Self and the heart of leadership through a screen that doesn't listen back. In Part II of this book, we'll share details of the new and improved "It starts with you . . .", which has been renamed as the dimension of Self with five distinct and defined attributes. But don't skip ahead, there's more to know about how the theory evolved!

Measurement: Take a "leadership selfie" to get a snapshot of your Human-Centered Leadership in Healthcare strengths

When I (Lucy, here) was in my PhD program, we had an entire course on instrument development, validation, psychometric analysis, and testing. Sounds fun, right? We learned everything and I mean everything that could be learned about instruments. While I absorbed a lot from my professors at the Medical University of South Carolina in 2009, this course was, quite honestly, not ranked very high on my own Likert scale of 1 to 5 with 1 = "Snooze Fest. Is it over yet?" 😴; 2 = "Meh, it's okay sometimes" 🤷‍♀️; 3 = "Not bad, has its moments" 😌; 4 = "Pretty fun, I actually look forward to it!" 😃; and 5 = "Best class ever! Can't wait to put this into practice!" 🎉. It's only taken more than 10 years to realize that I would now rate it a 5. At the time, I was trying my best to understand psychometrics, which can be a very challenging specialty of science to grasp. It took time and practical application to truly embrace the value of psychometrics as a field of science. Years have passed, and I'm now the first one to nerd out and ask for the evidence to illustrate that scales really measure what they say they'll measure and that they do it consistently. The importance of validated instruments, scales, and tools cannot be overemphasized. These tools are the foundation for science and evidence in healthcare. There are validated instruments that measure nearly every concept you can think of in healthcare: depression, anxiety, quality of life, pain, cognitive function, functional status, burnout, well-being, stress, sleep, delirium, risk for falls, self-compassion, healthy work environment, patient experience, attitudes toward disabled people, attitudes toward caring for those at the end of life, and so on. You get it, right? Validated tools help us measure whether our interventions are effective or in the case of screening tools, alert us to the risk of disease. To remember the importance of this, remember it's the "so what?" part of care or innovation. Whether it's an evidence-based practice project or an Institutional Review Board-approved research project, validated instruments are the gold standard to measure your outcome. Please don't confuse outcome metrics with process metrics. Process metrics are things like audits for compliance with a particular intervention such as bundled care in the ICU. The outcome measure is the "so what?", which would be something like reduced delirium in the ICU example. Our Magnet, Pathway, Beacon, Prism, and Lantern colleagues will thank us for sharing this distinction. Next, we'll share our "so what?" instrument that measures the four dimensions of HCL-HC and how it was developed from our original research using constructivist grounded theory.

From Theory to Instrument to Validation. The journey from theory to validated instrument is just that, a journey with planned stops and starts as well as unplanned detours. There are generally three steps (or stops) in the itinerary of instrument development: item development, scale development, and psychometric evaluation (Boateng, Neilands, Frongillo, Melgar-Quinonez, & Young, 2018). The following is an overview of these three steps that occurred from 2021 to 2024.

Item Development: Based on Research and Theoretical Construction. The HCL-HC theory was developed using constructivist grounded theory, which honors co-creation between participants, researchers, literature, and historical perspectives. As noted in our original research published in 2021, the aim was to identify and explore the attributes of nurse leaders who effectively balance human-centered needs with positive patient outcomes and operational metrics (Leclerc, Kennedy, & Campis, 2021). Through multiple focus groups with 39 nurses in various leadership roles, 15 attributes were identified and categorized into three dimensions: Awakener, Connector, and Upholder. These dimensions were linked to potential outcomes such as cultures of excellence, trust, and caring. The original 15 items for the HCL-HC self-assessment were inductively generated through qualitative, constructivist research using the central source of the voice of nurse leaders (Leclerc et al., 2021; Morgado, Meireles, Neves, Amaral, & Ferreira, 2017). The resulting self-assessment comprised 15 items with five items in each of the three dimensions of Awakener, Connector, and Upholder. The assessment responses were framed within a 5-point Likert scale with the following instructions: Each statement provides a possible strategy for leadership. Rate each statement on a scale of 1 to 5, indicating how likely you are to use this strategy. Answer as you actually conduct yourself. 5 = Always; 4 = Usually; 3 = Sometimes; 2 = Rarely; and 1 = Never. The questions were arranged in random order without identification of the specific dimension associated with each question (Podsakoff, Mackenzie, Lee, & Podsakoff, 2003; Schell & Oswald, 2013).

Pilot Testing. We conducted a pilot study with 60 datasets to evaluate the instrument's psychometric properties. The analysis revealed good factor loadings for 11 items, supporting construct and discriminant validity. Reliability testing showed Cronbach's alpha values of 0.88, 0.66, and 0.80 for Awakener, Connector, and Upholder, respectively. Recommendations included reducing the complexity of individual items, i.e., those that did not load satisfactorily. For example, the Motivator, an attribute of the dimension of the Awakener, was modified from "I provide a safe environment for my team members to grow and expect accountability for individual growth plans" to "I establish a learning culture that leverages the power of the individual's intrinsic motivation." Also, based on the pilot psychometric results, in parallel with continued inquiry into theoretical evolution, we expanded the theory of HCL-HC to include the dimension of Self with five associated attributes: Well-Being, Self-Care, Self-Compassion, Self-Awareness, and Mindfulness (Kennedy, Leclerc, & Campis, 2022; Leclerc, Kennedy, & Campis, 2023; Leclerc & Pabico, 2023; Leclerc et al., 2022). This resulted in a 20-item assessment with five items in each of the four dimensions. Also, based on recommendations by the third-party psychometrician who assisted with statistical analysis, the items for each dimension were grouped and headers were added for each dimension (Healthcare Environment, 2021).

Psychometric Testing. From there, data collection of the revised self-assessment continued from June 2021 to November 2023. A third-party psychometrician evaluated the updated 20-item self-assessment, which included 729 respondents and used exploratory factor analysis to assess construct validity (Healthcare Environment, 2023). The analysis revealed factor loadings greater than 0.40 for most items, though some items required further refinement. Reliability testing showed Cronbach's alpha values ranging from 0.662 to 0.766. Despite some challenges with the factor structure, the instrument demonstrated adequate reliability and validity. The Self subscale emerged as a distinct and predictive component, indicating that leaders who focus on Self are more effective in then providing an outward focus to Awaken, Connect, and Uphold their teams.

Discussion. The HCL-HC Assessment, now a 20-item scale with two factors (Awakener/Connector and Upholder), explains a significant portion of the variance in HCL-HC. The Self subscale, a separate five-item subscale, also demonstrated predictive validity related to the outward-facing dimensions. These findings support the theory that effective HCL begins with a focus on Self. The validated instrument provides a valuable tool for assessing and developing leadership qualities in healthcare settings, ultimately contributing to improved patient outcomes and organizational performance. Please refer to Appendix C for the updated definitions of the 20 attributes.

What's next?

- **Ongoing evolution of the theory**: The fact that Self is loaded as a unique subscale strengthens the understanding of how the four dimensions of HCL-HC relate to one another. We now understand, from these results, that Self supports the other three dimensions as we found Self is predictive of the outward focusing dimensions of Awakener, Connector, and Upholder. We will continue to

Would you like to use the assessment in your research or evidence-based practice project?

If you'd like to use the HCL-HC self-assessment, observer-direct report version, or observer-colleague version, please reach out to us at uLeadership®: team@uleadership.com. We'd love to collaborate with you on your research or translational science project. The assessment is free and all we request is that you share your results with us so we can advance the science!

Would you like to take the assessment for your own knowledge and awareness? Here's the link to the free, online HCL-HC self-assessment. You'll receive immediate results via email. https://www.uleadership.com/assessment/

PRO TIP

Process Measure

A process measure evaluates the methods and procedures used in delivering an intervention or innovation. It focuses on the actions taken during the delivery of an intervention, ensuring that the right steps are followed to achieve desired outcomes.

- Clinical examples include adherence to hand hygiene protocols or the frequency of blood pressure monitoring in hypertensive patients.
- HCL-HC examples include the number of leadership development sessions attended during an HCL-HC Essentials course or participant feedback on the relevance and impact of the training sessions or the implementation rate of new leadership practices introduced during training.

Outcome Measure

An outcome measure assesses the results of an intervention or innovation. It focuses on the end results, such as changes in health, quality of life, patient satisfaction, or leadership behaviors.

- Clinical examples include the rate of hospital readmissions, patient mortality rates, improvement in symptoms, or patient-reported quality of life.
- HCL-HC examples include outcomes resulting from the integration of HCL-HC: nurse retention, nurse leader retention, nurse engagement, patient experience, and quality metrics.

Both types of measures are essential for evaluating and improving the quality of healthcare services and leadership. Process measures evaluate progress toward the outcome, while outcome measures assess the ultimate effectiveness of the intervention or innovation.

explore how the Self influences the outward-facing dimensions and other metrics such as cultures of excellence, trust, and caring.

- **Ongoing exploration of predictive validity**: We will continue to determine predictive variables that support the development of a human-centered leader through continued inquiry and psychometric testing.
- **Ongoing revision of the instrument**: We plan to reduce complexity and evaluate the wording of the two items that did not load satisfactorily.

- **Ongoing data collection**: We're planning our next psychometric evaluation at 400 to 500 assessments (Morgado et al., 2017). One limitation of a large sample size, such as the 729 we had for the most recent analysis, is that it can lead to statistical significance for even very small, practically insignificant effects, essentially "overpowering" the analysis or resulting in "over-significance." This was a lesson we learned and want to share with others. It's a common rule of thumb that there should be at least 10 participants for each item on the scale, making an ideal of 15:1 or 20:1 (Morgado et al., 2017; Sveinbjornsdottir & Thorsteinsson, 2008).
- **Translation**: Currently, we're collaborating with a PhD nursing student in Portugal to translate the instrument into Portuguese. Stay tuned for more to come as we work to make the instrument accessible to our shared global community.

Mindset and Language: The Essence of Each Dimension

The benefit of time and real-world experience with nurses across the country and the world brought with it clarity related to the essence of each of the four dimensions of HCL-HC. The theory now clearly identifies a specific *mindset* and *language* for each dimension. You'll learn a lot more about each of the mindsets and languages, as well as examples of each, in the chapters dedicated to each dimension. But, for now, let's review how these changes came about.

As stated previously, as we worked with nurses to implement and integrate HCL-HC into real-world environments, the dimension of Self presented itself, front and center, as the foundation of effective leadership in complex healthcare environments. As you'll recall that whole "It starts with you . . ." part of leadership was not clearly defined in the original conceptualization. Working side-by-side with nurses and teams, the dimension of Self matured into a clearly defined *mindset of well-being*, where the leader prioritizes their own health and self-care. Effective teams recognized that having a leader who prioritizes well-being set the tone for how they could do the same. Along with the mindset, a language to illustrate the essence of Self arose from the nurses we worked with. They either lamented the fact that they didn't feel as if they mattered, or they confidently felt that they did matter in their organization. As you might guess, culture and environment influenced each of those viewpoints. The *language* associated with Self became positively framed as "*I Matter*," which reinforces the idea that taking care of oneself is essential to effectively care for others. By acknowledging their own needs and valuing their own health, leaders set a positive example for their teams and create a culture where self-nurturing is respected and encouraged.

The dimension of the Awakener focuses on inspiring and motivating others to achieve their best to nurture a culture of trust. As we worked with nurses who identified more strongly with the Awakener, it became clear that the *mindset* was one of *seeking excellence*, not only in their own work but also in the development of their team members. The Awakeners identified that there was a language associated with feeling sure in both themselves and others. The *language* of *"I believe in you"* is central to this dimension, as it conveys trust and confidence in others' abilities. There's a lot of power and weight in those words. Nurses shared that you can't just say that to someone and then walk away. The leader has a responsibility to back up *"I believe in you"* with actions such as mentoring, coaching, motivating, advocating, and crafting an environment to nurture excellence in everyone. By expressing belief in their team's potential, leaders empower individuals to strive for excellence, fostering a supportive environment where everyone is encouraged to grow and succeed.

As a Connector, the leader aims to bring unity to the community while crafting a culture of trust. The Connectors we encountered shared how being vulnerable and collaborative were central to their success in nurturing mutual trust. They recognized that when they embodied a consistent *mindset* of *not needing to have all the answers*, collective wisdom often led to the best outcomes. The reason for having diverse teams is to harness the power of strengths! When the leader can hand over "power" and stop micromanaging decisions, trust flourishes. The *language* of *"I trust you"* is pivotal here, as it signifies a willingness to rely on the expertise and judgment of others. As with any statement as compelling as this, the leader must "walk the talk" and back up their words with actions. These include being a collaborator, supporter, edgewalker, engineer, and authentic communicator. This approach builds strong, collaborative relationships within the team, promoting a culture of mutual respect, shared responsibility, and trust.

The dimension of the Upholder recognizes the humanity in self and others to co-create a culture of caring. As we collaborated with Upholders, it became evident that their superpower lies in the consistent and mindful approach to both individuals and the collective team, driven by a *mindset* of *inclusion*. This approach is characterized by a commitment to recognizing the value of every team member and fostering an inclusive environment. Leaders with this mindset actively seek to create an environment where everyone feels seen, heard, and cared for. The *language* of *"I see you"* is fundamental to this dimension of leadership, as it acknowledges the unique contributions and perspectives of each individual. To back up the language of "I see you," the leader is mindfully present, others-oriented, emotionally aware, socially and organizationally aware, and models personal wellness and health. By fostering an inclusive atmosphere, leaders ensure that diverse voices are valued and that everyone has a sense of belonging within the organization (Figure 1).

Trivium: Being-Knowing-Doing

trivium (noun) /trIv.i.əm/
(Latin): A place where three roads meet.
Figurative: A crossroads for knowledge, decision-making, or divergent paths.

As the minutes, days, months, and years passed, our work with boots-on-the-ground leaders provided fertile soil for the seeds of transformation to name the process we were seeing. This whole "it starts with you . . ." idea made sense to so many leaders, but, as you're aware, it's not been the prevailing way of thinking about leadership and development. Traditional leadership and educational models start with the idea that we need to obtain knowledge first (*Know*), then experientially develop competence (*Do*), and finally, use reflection to hardwire the skill or knowledge into our way of being (*Be*; Drake & Burns, 2004; Snook, Nohria, & Khurana, 2012; Styron, 2013). As we started to implement the theory in practice settings through leadership development programs, at first, we tried to apply this traditional educational model, but it kept feeling like trying to fit a square peg into a round hole. Something was off. Our team came together to reflect, in real time, on what the core issue could be. Why did *knowledge* not seem like the right first step? Why would the traditional model identify *being* as the final step? In the traditional model, why were the three practices mutually exclusive when it seems some would overlap? Guess what we did next? We went to the literature! We explored to see if there was a different way to think about transformative processes, a way that aligned with the idea of "it starts with you . . ." As expected, we identified several sources that resonated with our experiences. These sources included historical and contemporary ones, some centered on leadership, others on education, and a few that bridged both areas (Hesselbein & Shinseki, 2004; Tierney, 2021; United States Army, 1999). Our hunch was that the order of transformation started with *Being* and that the three concepts were interlocking and couldn't exist in isolation.

The Army and Diamonds. Let's start with the United States Army and the metaphor of diamonds. Did you know that the leadership framework for the Army is *Be, Know, Do*—character, knowledge, and action (United States Army, 1999)? This model, introduced in 1999, has persisted as the central way of teaching leadership to our nation's

FIGURE 1
Mindset and language of each dimension of HCL-HC.

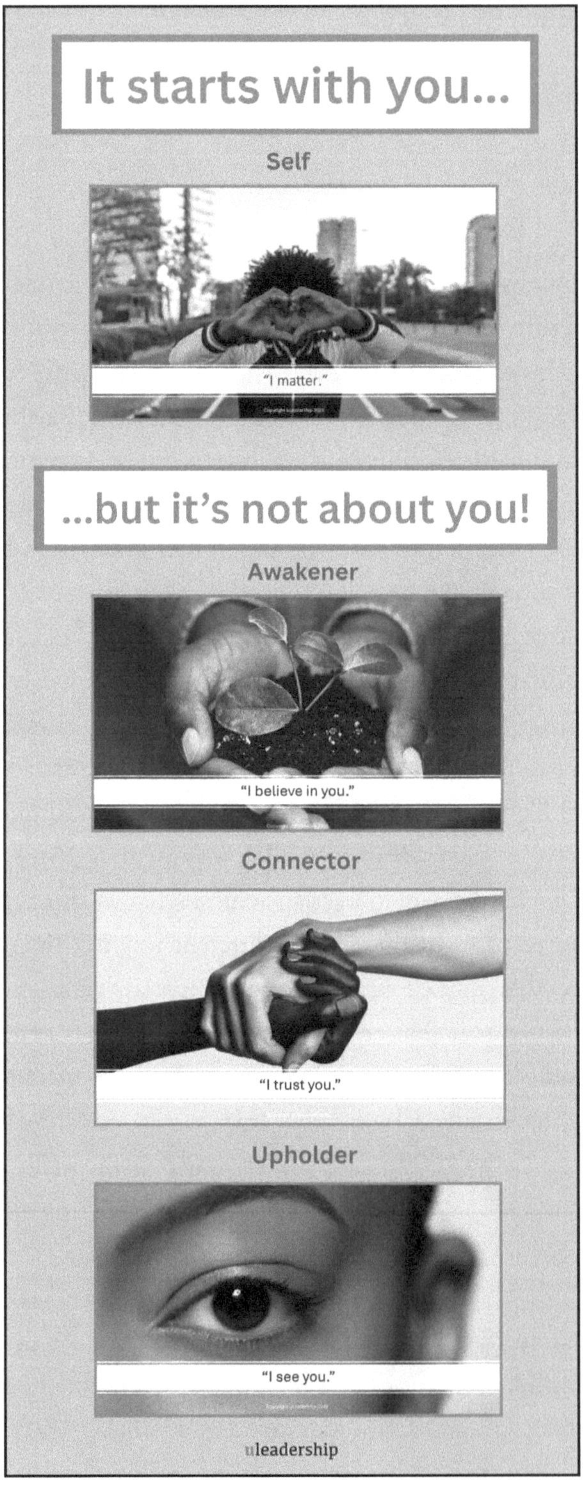

Army leaders: officers and non-commissioned officers, military and civilian, active and reserve. It was eye-opening to consider the longevity of the idea that character, values, and purpose (*Be*) are the first and most important attributes of leaders. And that the human dimension of "it starts with you . . ." is the foundation for being able to then outwardly focus on leading teams into often complex, chaotic, and conflicted situations. The words of General Edward C. Meyer, Former Army Chief of Staff, use the metaphor of a diamond to illustrate the linearity of the concepts of *Be, Know, Do.*

> Just as the diamond requires three properties for its formation—carbon, heat, and pressure—successful leaders require the interaction of three properties—character, knowledge, and application. Like carbon to the diamond, character is the basic quality of the leader. . . . But as carbon alone does not create a diamond, neither can character alone create a leader. The diamond needs heat. Man needs knowledge, study, and preparation. . . . The third property, pressure—acting in conjunction with carbon and heat—forms the diamond. Similarly, one's character, attended by knowledge, blooms through application to produce a leader.
>
> —General Edward C. Meyer
> Former Army Chief of Staff

Education + Leadership = Inclusivity. We also discovered the more recent work of Dr. Stephen Tierney, an expert on leadership in learning and academic environments with over 30 years of experience in the field. Tierney (2021) published a book merging the concepts of leadership and education. The premise of the book is similar to the Army's leadership philosophy of *Be, Know, Do*, but Tierney extends the reach of this methodology into education at all levels from the direct point of teaching to executive levels of academic leadership. He departs somewhat from the Army's approach by identifying the interconnectedness of the three concepts; they are mutually *inclusive* rather than exclusive or linear. What struck us most about Tierney's framework was the alignment between the theory of HCL-HC and the inclusivity of how the three "roads" of *Be-Know-Do* intersect into a trivium. Also, the basic definitions of each concept felt familiar and aligned with what we were witnessing in practice.

Being: Purpose and introspection
Knowing: Specialism and strategy
Doing: Implementation, networking, guardianship (ownership), and expertise

The View Through the Telescope Becomes Clear. As our team read through the literature and then collectively reflected through iterative comparative analysis with our real-world experiences, we developed a framework specific to HCL-HC. A framework that clearly and logically represented the way to operationalize the theory in a real-world setting. Honoring the time and space to pause and make good use of our proverbial telescope, we were able to name the essence of how to learn or strengthen the four dimensions of HCL-HC. Refer to Figure 2 for our framework, which we credit as an adaptation of Tierney's (2021) work. Also, as you read through the proceeding chapters, we'll dive deeper into how to apply the framework through each of the four dimensions of Self, Awakener, Connector, and Upholder.

The Work Continues: You Can't Just Drop the Mic

Over the past few years, the publications and presentations on HCL-HC have significantly contributed to the field, offering a comprehensive framework for leadership that prioritizes the well-being of both leaders and their teams. These publications, including peer-reviewed articles and influential books, have provided valuable insights and practical tools for implementing HCL-HC in various healthcare settings (See Ap-

FIGURE 2
Framework for operationalization of Human-Centered Leadership in Healthcare: *Being-Knowing-Doing*. Adapted from Tierney (2021).

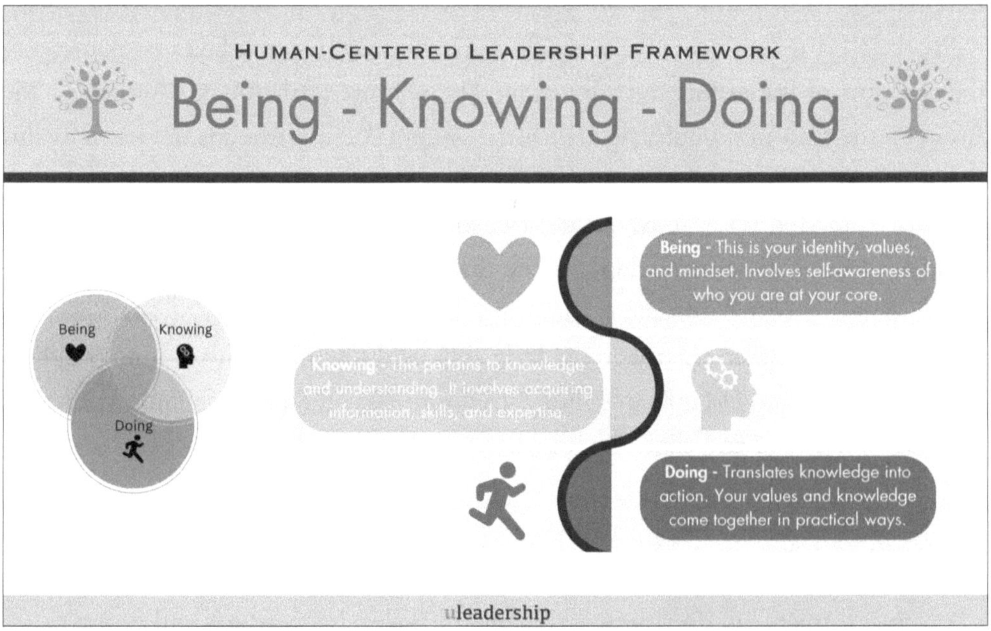

pendix A for a list of publications from 2020 to 2024). Also, the work has been presented at international, national, regional, and local conferences. Many of these were peer-reviewed:

- American Nurses Credentialing Center Magnet & Pathway™ Conference®
- ANA Enterprise Research Symposium
- Association for Leadership Science in Nursing Annual International Conference
- American Organization of Nurse Leaders Annual Conference
- International Council of Nursing Conference
- American Association of Colleges of Nursing Doctoral Education Conference
- Sigma Creating Healthy Work Environments Annual Conference
- International Association for Human Caring Annual Conference

Also, many presentations were invited keynotes. All that to say, the theory's emphasis on the four dimensions—Self, Awakener, Connector, and Upholder—has resonated with healthcare professionals globally, leading to widespread adoption and adaptation of its principles.

However, developing a seminal theory is just the beginning. Continuous validation and expansion of the theory are crucial to ensure its relevance and effectiveness in an ever-evolving healthcare landscape. As researchers and practitioners, we must persistently and rigorously test the theory's constructs and outcomes, gathering empirical evidence to support its claims. Additionally, expanding the theory to address emerging challenges and incorporating feedback from diverse healthcare environments will help refine and strengthen its application. We're taking cues from Copernicus and Einstein to keep listening and being open to new information that will only strengthen and make the theory better. This ongoing process of validation and expansion ensures that HCL-HC remains a dynamic and impactful approach to leadership in healthcare.

Global Connections: Humans Are Humans Wherever You Might Be In The World!
HCL-HC has achieved remarkable global reach, with researchers from diverse countries integrating its principles into their work. Scholars from China, Finland, Brazil, Spain, Germany, India, Italy, Argentina, England, Canada, Australia, New Zealand, Malaysia, Pakistan, Egypt, and the United States cite this approach in their research, writing, and projects. This widespread adoption underscores the universal appeal and

applicability of HCL-HC, as it resonates with the core values and needs of healthcare professionals worldwide.

Also, the influence of HCL-HC extends beyond the healthcare sector, illustrating its relevance to the common shared human experience. Researchers in various fields such as tourism and the film industry are recognizing the value of the four dimensions—Self, Awakener, Connector, and Upholder—in fostering effective leadership and healthier work environments.

This global and cross-disciplinary interest highlights the versatility and impact of HCL. Whether in healthcare or other sectors, the principles of prioritizing Self and focusing outward on others through the actions of Awakener, Connector, and Upholder are proving to be valuable. This approach not only enhances individual and team performance but also fosters a culture of empathy, collaboration, and inclusion, making it a powerful tool for leaders across the globe. Please refer to Appendix B for an overview of current work that cites HCL-HC.

Bringing It All Together

The evolution of HCL-HC over the past five years has been both profound and innovative. One pivotal advancement was the recognition of "Self" as a distinct dimension, expanding the framework beyond the original three dimensions of Awakener, Connector, and Upholder. This addition not only deepened the theory but also emphasized the foundational importance of a leader's relationship with themselves as the starting point for meaningful leadership. To further ground this theoretical expansion, a validated instrument was developed, enabling the assessment of all four dimensions from multiple perspectives—Self-Assessment, Others (Direct Reports), and Colleagues. This instrument has provided leaders with actionable insights into their leadership practices, promoting self-awareness and growth while strengthening relational dynamics within their teams.

Additionally, the past five years have seen the emergence of a unified mindset and language that encapsulate the essence of the four dimensions, fostering a shared understanding of HCL. Building on this foundation, a generative roadmap—focused on Being, Knowing, and Doing—has offered leaders tangible guidance for both personal and professional evolution. This roadmap has brought the four dimensions to life through actionable strategies, aligning leadership practices with the principles of relational leadership. A connecting theme has also emerged, highlighting the interplay between a leader's relationship with themselves and their relationships with others. This dual focus has solidified HCL as a dynamic and integrative approach, capable of addressing the complex needs of contemporary healthcare environments. As the theory continues to evolve, its emphasis on relational leadership and personal growth promises to shape the future of healthcare leadership in meaningful and lasting ways.

Discussion Questions for Groups

1. **Validation and Expansion of Seminal Theories**: Why is it important to continuously validate and expand seminal theories such as HCL-HC? How can ongoing research and practical application help refine and strengthen these theories over time?
2. **Global Integration of HCL**: How has the global reach of HCL-HC influenced its adoption and adaptation in different cultural contexts or even in different settings such as hospitals versus clinics? What are some examples of how researchers from various countries have integrated these principles into their work?
3. **Metaphors in Leadership Communication**: How does the metaphor of a hospital's physical architecture help illustrate the importance of the human aspect in healthcare? In what ways can metaphors be effective in communicating complex ideas and principles in leadership and other fields?

Reflection Questions for Individuals

1. Reflect on your own openness to change as it relates to research, healthcare environments, and new ways of thinking. Consider the evolution of HCL-HC as an example. Initially, this approach may have seemed revolutionary or even challenging to traditional leadership models.

2. Ask yourself: How willing are you to embrace new ideas and adapt to evolving practices in your field? Are you open to integrating innovative leadership concepts that prioritize well-being, trust, and inclusion? Reflect on how adopting a mindset of continuous learning and openness to change can enhance your professional and personal growth. How might these changes positively impact your interactions and relationships with others?

____

____

____

____

____

____

References

Ashcraft, S., Wilson, S., Nyström, K., Dusenbury, W., Wira, C., & Burrus, T. (2021). Care of the patient with acute ischemic stroke (prehospital and acute phase of care): Update to the 2009 comprehensive nursing care scientific statement: A scientific statement from the American Heart Association. *Stroke, 52* (5), e164–e178. doi: 10.1161/STR.0000000000000356

Boateng, G. O., Neilands, T. B., Frongillo, E. A., Melgar-Quinonez, H. R., & Young, S. L. (2018). Best practices for developing and validating scales for health, social, and behavioral research: A primer. *Frontiers in Public Health, 6*(149). doi: 10.3389/fpubh.2018.00149

Drake, S. M., & Burns, R. C. (2004). *Meeting standards through integrated curriculum.* Association for Supervision and Curriculum Development.

Healthcare Environment. (2021). Examination of psychometric properties and factor structure of the Human-Centered Leadership (HCL) in Healthcare Appraisal. May 5–9, 2021.

Healthcare Environment. (2023). Examination of psychometric properties and factor structure of the 20-item Human-Centered Leadership (HCL) Scale, an assessment of uLeadership, an expert organization in human centered leadership. December 10, 2023.

Hesselbein, F., & Shinseki, E. K. (2004). *Be-know-do: Leadership the army way (adapted from the official army leadership manual).* Jossey-Bass.

Morgado, F. F. R., Meireles, J. F. F., Neves, C. M., Amaral, A. C. S., & Ferreira, M. E. C. (2017). Scale development: Ten main limitations and recommendations to improve future research practices. *Psicologia, reflexao e critica: Revista semestral do Departamento de Psicologia da UFRGS, 30*(1). doi: 10.1186/s41155-016-0057-1

Podsakoff, P., MacKenzie, S., Lee, J., & Podsakoff, N. (2003). Common method biases in behavioral research: A critical review of the literature and recommended remedies. *Journal of Applied Psychology, 88*(5), 879–903.

Schell, K., & Oswald, F. (2013). Item grouping and item randomization in personality measurement. *Personality and Individual Differences, 55,* 317–321.

Snook, S., Nohria, N., & Khurana, R. (2012). *The handbook for teaching leadership: Knowing, doing, and being.* SAGE.

Styron, R. A. (2013). Interdisciplinary education: A reflection of the real world. *Systems, Cybernetics, and Informatics, 11*(9), 48–52.

Sveinbjornsdottir, S., & Thorsteinsson, E. B. (2008). Adolescent coping scales: A critical psychometric review. *Scandinavian Journal of Psychology, 49*(6), 533548. http://doi.org/10.1111/j.1467-9450.2008.00669.x

Tierney, S. (2021). *Leadership: Being, knowing, doing.* John Catt Publishing.

United States Army. (1999). *The U.S. army leadership field manual* (FM 22-100). Department of the Army. Retrieved from https://www.armyheritage.org/wp-content/uploads/2020/08/FM-22-100-Aug99.pdf

Recommended Reading

Campis, S., Kennedy, K., & Leclerc, L. (2022, July/August). Human-centered leadership in action: One turtle at a time. *Georgia Nursing, 83*(3), 9.

Campis, S., Kennedy, K., & Leclerc, L. (2022, Sept/Oct). Human-centered leadership in action: Embracing healthy boundaries. *Georgia Nursing, 82*(4), 6.

Campis, S., Leclerc, L., & Kennedy, K. (2024). Inspiring and nurturing Human-Centered Leaders: The vital role of mentorship. *Journal of Continuing Education in Nursing, 5,* 276–278.

Heier, C., Leclerc, L., Sanner-Stiehr, E., Busenhart, C., Park, S. H., & Nelson-Brantley, H. (2024). Improving nurse faculty job satisfaction: An action guide for academic nurse leaders. *Journal of Professional Nursing, 55,* 73–80.

Kennedy, K. (2024). Leadership style matters. *American Nurse, 19*(3), 48. doi: 10.51256/anj032448

Kennedy, K., Campis, S., & Leclerc, L. (2020). Human-centered leadership: Creating change from the inside out. *Nurse Leader, 18*(3), 227–231. doi: 10.1016/j.mnl.2020.03.009

Kennedy, K., Leclerc, L., & Campis, S. (2021a). *Human-centered leadership in healthcare: Evolution of a revolution.* Morgan James Publishing.

Kennedy, K., Leclerc, L., & Campis, S. (2021b). *Shifts, the journal for nurses, by nurses.* Morgan James Publishing.

Kennedy, K., Leclerc, L., & Campis, S. (2022). The great realization: Nurses are in the driver's seat. *Nurse Leader, 20*(5), 480–484. doi: 10.1016/j.mnl.2022.05.011

Kennedy, K., Leclerc, L., & Campis, S. (2023). Human-centered leadership. In J. J. Fitzpatrick & C. M. Alfes (Eds.), *Nurse leadership and management: Foundations for executive administration* (pp. 552–554). Springer Publishing.

Leclerc, L., Bailey, K. D., Fitzpatrick, J., Kennedy, K., & Raso, R. (2023) Getting schooled in relational leadership. *Journal of Nursing Education, 62*(11), 599–600. doi: 10.3928/01484834-20231010-02

Leclerc, L., D'Aquino, V., Lance, L., & Poole, V. (2024). Blending science, technology, and humanity: The dynamic role of radiology nursing. *Journal of Radiology Nursing, 43*(4), 235–239.

Leclerc, L., & Hoffman, C. (2024, July/August). An exemplar in honoring the shared human experience: Nurse honor guards. *Georgia Nursing, 84*(3), 5.

Leclerc, L., Kennedy, K., & Campis, S. (2020). Human-centered leadership in health care: An idea that's time has come. *Nursing Administration Quarterly, 44*(2), 117–126.

Leclerc, L., Kennedy, K., & Campis, S. (2021). Human-centered leadership in health care: A contemporary nursing leadership theory generated via constructivist grounded theory. *Journal of Nursing Management, 29*(2), 294–306. doi: 10.1111/jonm.13154

Leclerc, L., Kennedy, K., & Campis, S. (2023). Cultural intelligence (CQ): Flex your CQ muscle through a human-centered leadership workout! *Nurse Leader, 21*(3), 362–365.

Leclerc, L., & Pabico, C. (2023). A blueprint for well-being: Modeling the way through Human-Centered Leadership and Pathway to Excellence. *Nursing Management, 54*(4), 9–16. doi: doi10.1097/01.NUMA.0000921892.27917.78

Leclerc, L., Strenge-McNabb, K., Thibodeaux, T., Campis, S., & Kennedy, K. (2022). Relational leadership: A contemporary and evidence-based approach to improve nursing work environments. *Nursing Management, 53*(7), 24–34. doi: doi10.1097/01.NUMA.0000834580.84896.55

Lesandrini, J., & Leclerc, L. (2024). Fostering excellence in healthcare: The imperative for ethical leadership training in nurse leaders. *Nurse Leader, 22*(3), 273–277.

Raso, R., Bailey, K. D., Fitzpatrick, J., Kennedy, K., & Leclerc, L. (2024). Bold inquiry into relational leadership. *Nursing Management, 55*(1), 7–8. doi: 10.1097/nmg.0000000000000085

PART II

It Starts with You—The Dimension of Self

Before leaders can inspire others, they must first understand themselves—and that begins with clarity of purpose, a commitment to well-being, and the belief that "I matter." In this part, we explore how defining your "why" serves as an anchor, guiding decisions, and shaping leadership with intention. But purpose alone isn't enough—sustaining leadership requires prioritizing well-being, and recognizing that self-care isn't selfish, it's foundational to showing up fully for others. At the core of Human-Centered Leadership in Healthcare is the language of "I matter"—a simple but profound shift that reinforces self-worth, resilience, and the ability to lead with authenticity. When leaders embrace these three ideas, they move beyond simply functioning in a system—they begin to reshape it from the inside out, leading with presence, purpose, and balance.

CHAPTER 3

The Importance of Knowing Our "Why"

The two most important days in your life are the day you are born and the day you find out why.

—Mark Twain, American writer, humorist, and essayist

In a small village nestled between the mountains, there lived a young artist named Leo. Leo was known for his exceptional skill in creating beautiful pottery, yet he often felt something was missing. He could never shake off the feeling that his work lacked true purpose.

One day, an old traveler visited the village and admired Leo's pottery. The traveler asked, "Why do you create these beautiful pieces, young man?"

Leo hesitated, unsure how to respond. "I don't know," he said. "I suppose I just do it because I can."

The traveler smiled and said, "Understanding the 'why' behind what we do gives our actions meaning and direction. Without it, we may produce beautiful things, but we miss out on a deeper fulfillment."

Inspired by the traveler's words, Leo embarked on a journey of self-discovery. He traveled far and wide, learning about diverse cultures, their stories, and how they used pottery to connect with their heritage and express their identity. Along the way, he met people who used pottery to preserve their history, pass down traditions, and bring communities together.

When Leo returned to his village, he felt a renewed sense of self-awareness and purpose. He realized that his craft wasn't just about creating beautiful pieces; it was about expressing himself through storytelling, preserving memories, and connecting with people. With this newfound understanding, Leo's pottery took on a deeper significance, and his work became more meaningful and fulfilling.

Leo's journey of self-discovery taught him the importance of understanding his "why." It gave him a purpose that transformed his work and enriched his life, reminding us that knowing our purpose can lead to greater fulfillment and impact.

Nursing, much like art, blends technical skill with creativity, empathy, and a deep understanding of the human experience. Just as an artist carefully selects their tools and techniques to create something meaningful, nurses use their knowledge, intuition, and compassion to tailor care to each individual's unique needs.

Both nursing and art involve storytelling—whether it's through a painting that conveys emotion or through listening to and understanding patients' stories to provide holistic care. Nurses, like artists, must be adaptable and resourceful, responding to ever-changing circumstances and finding innovative solutions.

Moreover, both fields are profoundly human. They require a connection with others, the ability to see beauty and possibility even in challenging situations, and a dedication to making a difference in the world. In this way, nursing transcends routine tasks and becomes a form of artistry—one that transforms lives.

Human-Centered Leadership in Healthcare (HCL-HC) begins with understanding our "why." Our why is not solely about what we do or how we do it, but rather the inspiration and motivation that drives our actions and decisions. Understanding the purpose and why behind our behaviors and actions helps us gain insight into our values and motivations. This self-awareness allows us to make more informed and deliberate choices because we are better able to evaluate options and understand consequences. Let's reflect on Leo's story. Initially, Leo created pieces without understanding the true purpose behind his work. It was only after receiving advice from a wise traveler that Leo embarked on a journey to discover the deeper meaning of his craft. Leo's art reflected his value of storytelling, honoring memories, and connecting with others and this became his why.

Reflecting on our actions and decisions supports our ability to identify areas for personal growth and development. When we are in a state of being that is connected to our why, we have the opportunity to live a more intentional, authentic, and fulfilling life.

Understanding our why in healthcare leadership starts with recognizing our core values. In what ways do our personal values influence how we lead and engage as healthcare professionals? Let's begin by defining the concept of values. Values are our core beliefs that serve as guiding principles for our behavior, decisions, and actions. They function as a moral compass, helping us discern right from wrong while shaping our attitudes and influencing how we conduct ourselves. Values fuel our motivation and passion, driving us to pursue our purpose with determination and enthusiasm. Values can be personal, organizational, or societal, often reflecting what is most important to us. Grasping the rationale behind our actions and decisions, much like Leo did with his craft, is essential. Both why and "purpose" explore the fundamental reasons and driving forces behind our actions. These closely intertwined concepts reflect the core motivations that shape and influence our behavior.

As Simon Sinek (2011) explains, if you don't know the why you can't know the "how." By consistently reflecting on our core values and motivations, we ensure that our leadership remains empathetic, patient-focused, and aligned with our goal of improving lives, by encouraging (I believe in you), supporting (I trust you), and inspiring (I see you) others to become their best selves. When we understand our purpose and the reasons behind our actions, it becomes much easier to navigate challenges and remain steadfast in pursuing goals. This clarity fuels our inner drive, empowering us to step outside our comfort zone, embrace risks, and unlock personal growth and achievement.

Deepening Your Why: Powerful Reflection Questions for Meaningful Insights

- What activities or experiences bring you a deep sense of fulfillment or joy?
- How do your values align with the way you live your life? Are there areas where they don't align?
- What legacy do you hope to leave behind, and how does that shape your sense of purpose?
- How does your understanding of purpose evolve as you grow more self-aware?
- How do you react to constructive feedback, and what does it teach you about yourself?

This understanding empowers us to lead with authenticity, compassion, and a clear sense of purpose, creating a supportive and innovative healthcare environment.

Fueling Your Purpose: Why Well-Being Is the Key to Long-Term Impact

Once we've identified our purpose and the motivations behind it, it's equally vital to dedicate attention to building the foundation that enables us to actively and effectively pursue it. Let's look back at Leo's story. As Leo ventured deeper into his journey of purpose, he discovered another truth—that understanding one's purpose alone was not enough. To bring his vision to life and share his art meaningfully, he needed to understand himself and maintain his sense of well-being. He learned from other artists the importance of harmony—between their art and their mental, physical, and emotional health. Leo began to practice mindfulness and self-nurturing, ensuring he had the energy and clarity to pour his heart into his craft. He found that taking moments to rest, reflect, and connect with his inner self not only sustained his sense of purpose but also enriched it. Discovering his purpose was powerful, but sustaining the energy, passion, and clarity needed to live it out required focusing on his well-being.

Prioritizing our wellness and well-being isn't a deviation from our purpose—it's the foundation that keeps us aligned with it, empowering us to show up as the best version of ourselves. HCL-HC begins with the essential dimension of the "self," representing the leader as an "individual in the center." This dimension encompasses personal being, knowledge, values, behaviors, and the interplay between them.

Personal being refers to our core essence, including our identity, character, values, beliefs, and the intrinsic qualities that make us unique. It's about understanding who we are, what we stand for, and what motivates us. It's the foundation of who we are as a person, encompassing our thoughts, emotions, and experiences that shape our understanding of ourselves and the world around us. Our personal being is what makes us unique but also brings connection with others. Individual uniqueness is the distinct characteristics and traits that make each person different from everyone else. This uniqueness encompasses a wide range of attributes, including our personality, talents, beliefs, experiences, and values. These elements combine to create a personal and unique identity that shapes how we perceive the world, interact with others, and pursue our goals. Celebrating and understanding individual uniqueness fosters a sense of appreciation for diversity, encourages personal growth, and strengthens interpersonal relationships by recognizing the valuable contributions each person brings to a community. It's the combination of all the attributes that define an individual's true self. It's the holistic representation of a person.

Self-Awareness and the Art of Receiving Feedback

Self-awareness is a specific aspect of personal being. It involves an individual's conscious recognition and understanding of their own emotions, thoughts, values, strengths, and weaknesses. Self-awareness is about having insight into one's character and how it influences actions and interactions with others. Human-centered leaders understand that a strong sense of self-awareness is critical to effective leadership because it shapes how leaders understand themselves, regulate their emotions, interact with others, and pursue continuous growth. A keen sense of self-awareness also creates space for feedback on how behaviors are perceived by others. Feedback isn't always easy to hear, mainly because someone's feedback is sometimes criticism masked as feedback. We can feel on a primal level, the difference between the two. So, let's take a minute here to discuss the difference between feedback and criticism. Criticism can be perceived as harsh and negative and tends to focus on our faults and weaknesses. Many times, criticism is rooted in personal bias and preferences. When we are being criticized, we feel defensive, hurt, and sometimes helpless. Criticism is often seen as negative because it tends to carry a judgmental tone, which can feel personal or attacking. The word itself historically implies pointing out flaws or shortcomings, and people may associate it with disapproval or confrontation. This perception can make it harder to accept, even when it's well-intentioned. The way criticism is interpreted can depend on the tone, context, and relationship between the people involved, making it an incredibly potent part of communication.

Feedback, on the other hand, is framed as neutral or constructive (Erdeljac & Westrick, 2018). It is seen as a respectful and helpful way of communicating, focusing on improvement rather than fault-finding. Feedback is rooted in objective observations versus subjective interpretations. The term feedback also suggests a dialogue or exchange, emphasizing collaboration and mutual growth. This positive framing makes it feel less threatening and more actionable. It feels safe rather than hurtful. One framework for providing feedback is called the *Lighthouse Method* (Evanish, 2024).

A lighthouse and feedback share a striking similarity in their purpose: both aim to guide and illuminate paths to safety or improvement. Just as a lighthouse helps sailors find their way through uncertain waters, feedback provides individuals with direction, pointing them toward actions, decisions, or areas for growth. One framework for

Lighthouse Method for Providing Feedback

PREPARE	Collect examples Identify patterns Be specific about desired changes
LISTEN	Providing feedback is a conversation, not a "drive by" Listen for key information Ask appropriate questions
ACT	Be specific in your expectations Follow-up

Note: Adapted from Evanish (2024).

providing feedback is described as the Lighthouse Method and includes three specific actions.

In the end, the difference often lies in the delivery. Criticism that's specific, respectful, and solution-oriented is more likely to be received positively—essentially transforming into what we'd call feedback (Evanish, 2024). There's an emotional weight to the process of giving and receiving feedback. It often comes with an underlying vulnerability, which makes it a deeply human experience.

Human-centered leaders, with the help of feedback, recognize their strengths, weaknesses, values, intentions, and emotions. This awareness enables them to make informed decisions, communicate effectively, and navigate challenges with authenticity and integrity. Developing a strong sense of self-awareness doesn't happen overnight. It's an ongoing journey, enriched by daily practices of reflection, feedback, self-compassion, and mindfulness. This is why HCL-HC emphasizes "self" as the foundational dimension of leadership.

Discussion Questions for Groups

1. Purpose can shape the way leaders navigate challenges and inspire others, yet it often evolves over time. How has your sense of purpose changed throughout your leadership journey? What key moments or experiences helped refine your why, and how do you actively keep it at the center of your leadership decisions?
2. Receiving feedback can be a vulnerable process, but distinguishing helpful insights from harsh criticism is essential for growth. Reflect on a time when feedback significantly shaped your leadership approach. What strategies have

helped you receive feedback without defensiveness? How can leaders foster an environment where feedback feels constructive rather than threatening?

Reflection Questions for Individuals

1. How does knowing your why shape the way you care for yourself, and how do you currently balance purpose with well-being?

   ____

   ____

   ____

   ____

   ____

2. What habits help you stay aligned with your why while maintaining a healthy focus on self-care?

   ____

   ____

   ____

   ____

   ____

   ____

References

Erdeljac, P., & Westrick, C. (2018). Feedback and leadership—leadership in public health. In T. Huber, L. Brietenstine, L. Schreiber, K. Budzik, T. Moffitt, & J. Persol (Eds.), *Leadership lessons in healthcare and public health.* Pressbooks. Retrieved from https://ohiostate.pressbooks.pub/pubhhmp6615/chapter/challenges-and-obstacles/

Evanish, J. (2024). How to give constructive feedback to improve and motivate your team in 3 simple steps. *Lighthouse Blog.* Retrieved from https://getlighthouse.com/blog/give-constructive-feedback-motivate-improve

Sinek, S. (2011). *Start with why: How great leaders inspire everyone to take action.* Penguin Books.

Recommended Reading

Baker, A. B., Perreault, D., Reid, A., & Blanchard, C. M. (2013). Feedback and organizations: Feedback is good, feedback—friendly culture is better. *Canadian Psychology, 54*(4), 260–268.

Geisler, J. (2019, November). *Effective performance management requires knowing how to give positive feedback.* Healthcare Financial Management Association.

Geisler, J. (2019, December). *What leaders should know before having tough conversations about performance.* Healthcare Financial Management Association.

Johns Hopkins University. (2019). Why do I avoid giving feedback? Self-assessment. Retrieved from https://hr.jhu.edu/wp-content/uploads/2019/08/Why-Do-I-Avoid-Giving-Feedback.pdf.

Riegel, D. G. (2019, June 24). The assumptions employees make when they don't get feedback. *Harvard Business Review.* Retrieved from hbr.org/2019/06/the-assumptions-employees-make-when-they-dont-get-feedback

CHAPTER 4

The Mindset—"It Starts with Me"

Wellness is the complete integration of body, mind, and spirit—the realization that everything we do, think, feel, and believe affects our state of well-being.

—Greg Anderson, Author and Founder of the America Wellness Project

Wellness is more than just a state of health—it is the intricate balance of body, mind, and spirit, woven together by the choices we make every day. It is not a destination but a continuous process, much like tending a garden. Every thought we cultivate, every habit we nourish, and every belief we embrace shapes the landscape of our well-being. Just as a seed holds the potential for growth, so do we. In the same way that soil must be enriched, watered, and exposed to sunlight, we thrive when we nurture ourselves—through movement that strengthens, reflection that grounds us, and connections that uplift. True wellness is not perfection but the resilience to adapt, the willingness to tend to what needs care, and the patience to trust the process.

My grandmother was a gardener. In fact, I come from a family of gardeners—my mom, my aunt, my sisters, and my daughters all love being outside, hands in the dirt. I vividly remember my grandmother's yard, a vibrant oasis filled with azaleas, irises, hyacinths, geraniums, and her favorite, violets. She also had a small vegetable garden where she grew tomatoes and cucumbers in the summer and collard greens in the fall. Her pride and joy, though, was a large pecan tree that stood in the center of her yard.

During the summer, you could always find my grandmother tending to her garden early in the morning or late in the evening. Her house was never without fresh-cut flowers such as hydrangeas, gardenias, or jasmine, and she always seemed to find something new to plant. She had a knack for taking clippings of plants from places she visited, adding pieces of the world to her garden. Once, during a camping trip in the Smoky Mountains, she returned with a sack full of plant clippings (probably illegally). Some of them thrived; others didn't. But she always told me, "It's worth trying, even if not everything grows."

When I got married and moved into my first house, my grandmother gave me a clipping from her garden as a gift. I planted it in the small backyard garden I started, and 31 years later, that plant is still growing strong. Her passion for gardening taught me a lot about life. Just as a garden thrives with care and dedication, so do we. Cultivating a sense of well-being takes effort and intentionality. Over the years, I've learned many life lessons from gardening. One that stands out is the hidden potential in every seed. Seeds may be tiny, fragile, and covered by a tough shell, but when they're placed in a healthy environment and nurtured with water, sunlight, and care, the shell cracks open, and growth begins. What lies inside a seed isn't immediately visible, but the flower or fruit is already there, waiting to flourish.

The Gardener: It Really Does Start with You . . .

Similarly, our lives are full of possibilities. By nurturing our body, mind, and spirit, we can grow and bloom into our fullest potential. Like gardening, this requires preparation and care. For a garden to thrive, the soil must be healthy—it's the foundation. Before planting, a gardener must understand the soil: Is it sandy or clay? What's the pH? How does it retain water? Does it have the right nutrients? Healthy soil makes everything easier, while neglected soil leads to weeds and struggle.

This idea parallels our own lives. A healthy mindset is the foundation for a thriving self. When our thoughts are balanced and nourished, we flourish. Yet, as all gardeners know, even in healthy gardens, weeds exist. Surprisingly, some weeds aren't entirely bad—they can protect the soil from erosion, attract beneficial insects, and create pathways for worms. But when weeds grow unchecked, they steal nutrients, overshadow beauty, and can choke the life from a garden. In our lives, weeds might take the form of negative thoughts, emotions, or even toxic relationships. Left untended, they sap our energy and diminish our potential. Mindfulness, self-awareness, and self-compassion are the tools we use to remove these weeds and nurture growth.

Gardening also teaches patience and gratitude. In today's world of instant gratification, we've lost the joy of anticipation. Gardening reminds us that patience is a virtue. We wait for flowers to bloom, for plants to grow, for tomatoes to ripen, and then—almost as if by magic—it happens. It's a reminder that life unfolds in its own time.

Gardening keeps us grounded. It reminds us that we are part of a larger cycle, connected to something bigger. And, just like in the garden, when we show ourselves care and compassion, we grow, we blossom, and we thrive.

Gardening has always been a metaphor for life and growth, offering lessons about nurturing, patience, and balance. Just as tending a garden requires dedication and care, so does cultivating a sense of well-being in our lives. Through intentional effort and mindfulness, we can thrive, grow, and positively influence the world around us.

This idea aligns with the principles of Human-Centered Leadership in Healthcare (HCL-HC). At its core, Human-Centered Leadership (HCL) begins with the self—what Kennedy, Leclerc, and Campis (2022) refer to as "the leader" or "the human in the center." This essential dimension encompasses an individual's values, strengths, behaviors, and overall sense of well-being. Guided by the mindset, "It starts with me," this approach emphasizes personal responsibility and the understanding that we have the power to influence our own lives and environments.

Just as a gardener tends to the soil before planting, a leader nurtures their inner self to create a foundation for growth. "It starts with me" is not just a mindset but a way of being—rooted in self-awareness, authenticity, self-compassion, and mindfulness. By understanding our values, strengths, and weaknesses, we gain clarity about who we are and how we show up in the world. When we embrace our authentic selves, we act with consistency and purpose. When we show ourselves kindness and compassion, we foster fortitude and a growth mindset. And by being fully present in the moment, we uncover opportunities for growth and improvement.

Achieving a sense of well-being is a multidimensional journey. It involves harmonizing various aspects of life—physical health, mental and emotional stability, social connections, and a sense of purpose. True well-being is not simply the absence of stress or illness; it is the presence of positive emotions, fortitude, and life satisfaction. It requires caring for the "soil" of our lives: practicing mindfulness, managing stress, seeking support when needed, and fostering a healthy mindset.

Well-Being: Are You Tending Your Own Garden?

Like a thriving garden, our well-being flourishes when we address all dimensions of life. Financial stability provides peace of mind, intellectual curiosity stimulates growth, and spiritual connection nurtures the soul. By finding balance across these areas, we create a life that is both fulfilling and meaningful.

Human-centered leaders recognize the profound connection between well-being and effective leadership. Just as a healthy garden inspires those who see it, a leader with a strong sense of well-being positively impacts their team, organization, and community. Tools like the Wheel of Well-Being help us visualize and assess the various dimensions of our lives, guiding us to the areas that may need attention and celebrating the areas where we thrive.

Ultimately, caring for ourselves is not a sign of selfishness or weakness, but an act of strength. Our well-being is not only about us; it extends to the lives we touch and the difference we make. Whether we're nurturing a garden, ourselves, or those around us, the principles remain the same: With care, dedication, and intentionality, we can foster growth, resilience, and beauty. Now, it's your turn! Take a few minutes to do a self-assessment to see where your strengths and opportunities for well-being fall within the domains of the Wheel of Well-Being (Figure 3).

Self-Awareness: What Does Your Garden Look Like to Others or to Yourself?

Recognizing the self as the cornerstone in HCL is crucial, as it impacts how leaders comprehend themselves, regulate their emotions, interact with others, and pursue personal and professional growth. Self-awareness lies at the heart of this dimension. It involves acknowledging our values, thoughts, and intentions, and ensuring that our behaviors, the outward and visible actions, align with our personal principles.

Just as a gardener carefully examines the soil to understand its strengths and limitations, human-centered leaders strive to acknowledge their strengths, weaknesses, values, and intentions. This heightened self-awareness equips leaders to navigate challenges with clarity, make informed decisions, and communicate effectively. Interactions with others—like the relationships between plants in a garden—are influenced by our self-perception and how others perceive us. When these views align, connections flourish; when they diverge, communication and collaboration may falter. Internal self-awareness,

FIGURE 3

The Wheel of Well-Being.

Self—It starts with you!

The Wheel of Well-Being

Take a few minutes to rate yourself in each of the eight domains of well-being. Use the guided questions on the following page to inform your ratings.

Use the scale of 1 to 5 with these interval descriptions to guide you. You may fall somewhere in between on the scale.

5 = I've got this down to a science!

3 = I'm hit or miss with this one.

1 = I've got some work to do!

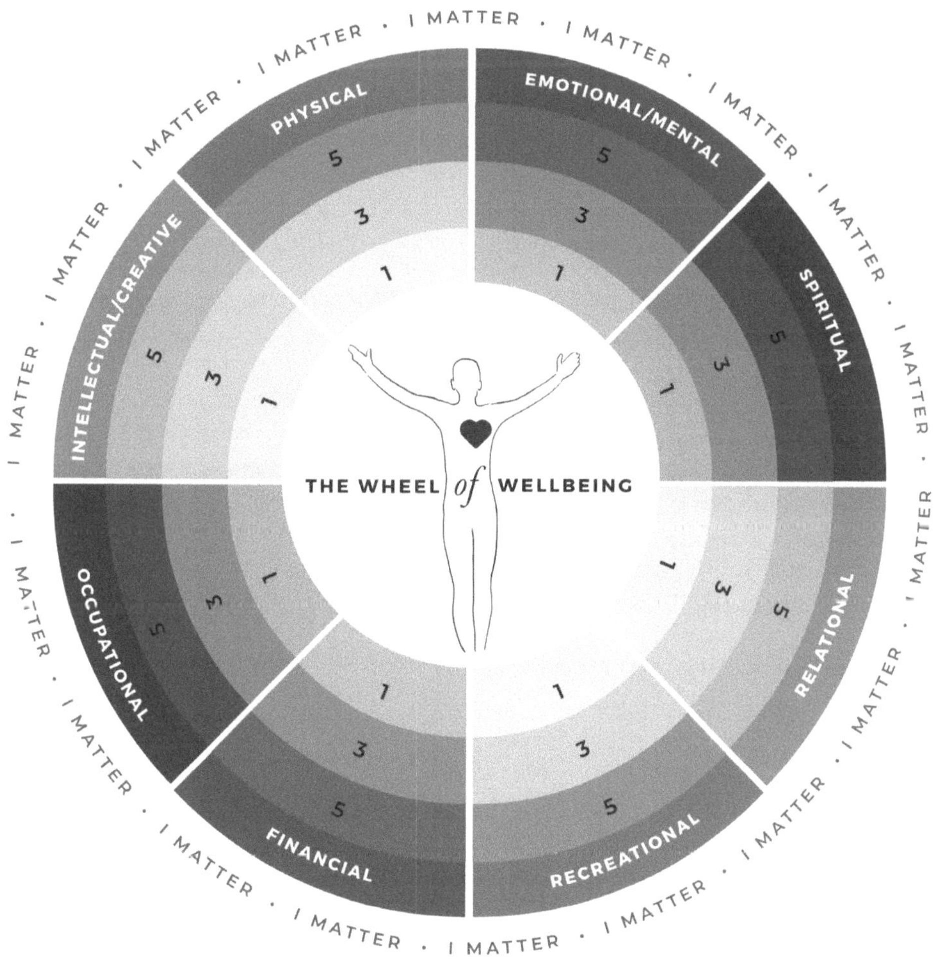

The Eight Domains of Health and Well-Being: Worksheet

In each of the eight domains, consider where you are today and where you would like to be. How will you move closer to your vision of health and wellness?

INTELLECTUAL/CREATIVE	PHYSICAL
Am I able to find ways to expand my knowledge and connect to my creativity? • I am a lifetime learner. • I use my creative abilities. • I read often. • I exercise critical thinking skills. • I have a positive self-image. • I focus on learning new skills.	Am I choosing things to nurture my body? • I exercise regularly. • I get seven to nine hours of sleep each night and feel rested in the morning. • I seek advice from healthcare professionals if I have a concern I can't solve on my own. • I avoid harmful use of drugs (over the counter, prescription, or illicit) • I drink alcohol responsibly. • I maintain healthy eating patterns with clean, whole foods like fruit and vegetables. • I stay hydrated and drink water throughout the day.
EMOTIONAL/MENTAL	**SPIRITUAL**
Am I able to cope effectively with life and build satisfying relationships with others? • I find healthy ways to cope with stress. • I ask for assistance when I need it, either from friends, family, or professionals. • I accept responsibility for my own actions. • I feel good about myself and believe others like me for who I am. • I treat myself with kindness and compassion. • I'm flexible and able to adapt to life's changes. • I can express all ranges of feelings and manage emotion-related behaviors in a healthy way. • I maintain a balance of work, friends, family, and other obligations. • I don't let my emotions get the better of me. I think before I act. • I have a healthy relationship with social media.	Am I able to understand and accept my connection to the world and my place in it? • I take time to think about what is important in my life—who I am, what I value, and where I fit in. • I make time for relaxation and reflection during the day. • I pray or meditate each day. • I have a belief system in place. • My values guide my decisions and actions. • I have a sense of purpose in my life, I understand my "why." • I'm tolerant and accepting of the views of others. • I'm active in communities and causes I care about. • I'm able to help others in need. • I work to create balance and peace with my interpersonal relationships, community, and the world.
RELATIONAL	**RECREATIONAL**
Am I able to develop and nurture relationships and a sense of belonging? • I focus on maintaining social connections by keeping in touch and staying connected with others. • I interact with a diverse group of friends.	Am I enjoying life and making it fun? • I spend time outdoors enjoying nature. • I take vacations or short getaways regularly. • I laugh every day. • I find time to relax every day.

RELATIONAL	RECREATIONAL
• I draw healthy boundaries with myself and others. I nurture positive and healthy relationships. • I have good communication skills. • I reach out to others for support and ask for help when I need it.	• I find time to be with friends and family on a regular basis. • I find ways to move my body every day.
FINANCIAL	**OCCUPATIONAL**
Am I satisfied with my current and future financial situations? • I'm comfortable with what I'm earning to satisfy my needs. • I maintain a budget and monitor my spending. • I explore ways to save money. • I'm financially responsible.	Am I receiving personal satisfaction and enrichment from my work? • I have career goals. • I'm satisfied with the work I do. • My work is meaningful to me. • I have good work habits and maintain harmony between work and life. • I'm able to learn from my mistakes and move forward.

understanding our inner workings, helps us stay true to ourselves and maintain balance, while external self-awareness enables us to recognize our impact on others and adapt our actions to build constructive relationships. In our previous book, *HCL-HC: Evolution of a Revolution*, we introduced a model and framework, developed by Joseph Luft and Harrington Ingram, called the Johari Window. This tool can be used by leaders and teams to enhance self-awareness, promote personal growth, and strengthen interpersonal relationships. We went a step further and created a HCL-HC Johari Window using dimensions, attributes, and associated leadership behaviors. The tool uses a four-quadrant grid to represent aspects of an individual's personality:

1. **Open**: Traits known to both the individual and others.
2. **Blind Spot**: Traits others perceive but the individual is unaware of.
3. **Hidden**: Traits known to the individual but kept private from others.
4. **Unknown**: Traits unknown to both the individual and others.

Understanding your Open, Hidden, Blind, and Unknown Self can be transformative. Take a moment to complete the exercise provided—how do your traits compare with others' perceptions?

Exercise: Exploring Your Johari Window Through the HCL Lens

Objective: Improve self-awareness and gain insights into how others perceive you.

Overview: To complete the activity, you need to choose words that you think describe you from a set list and get your peers to do the same. You then explore the differences between the words you and they chose. Once you understand where the differences are, you can create a plan to help you bridge the gap. The following steps will help you do this:

Step 1: Identify Your Traits

Use the following list of words/adjectives representing traits and attributes of a human-centered leader. Circle 5–10 that you believe belong in your **Open Self**.

Accepting	Adaptable	Bold	Advocate	Calm
Caring	Courageous	Wise	Mindful	Others-Oriented
Reflective	Dependable	Kind	Compassionate	Supportive
Empathetic	Patient	Innovative	Helpful	Warm
Creative	Optimistic	Inclusive	Trustworthy	Quiet
Cheerful	Confident	Spiritual	Observant	Safe
Humble	Outspoken	Motivating	Friendly	Collaborative
Empowering	Role Model	Edgewalker	Open-Minded	Micromanager
Authentic	Understanding	Competent	Capable	Growth Mindset
Present	Emotionally Aware	Authentic Communicator	Self-Compassionate	Personally Well and Healthy

Step 2: Get Feedback

Ask a few trusted friends, family members, or colleagues to select traits and attributes they associate with you from the same list. This could also be a team activity. Compare their selections with yours.

Step 3: Plot the Feedback

- Traits you both selected go into **Open**.
- Traits only they selected go in **Blind Spots**.
- Traits you listed but they didn't go in **Hidden**.
- Any new insights or unexpected traits may belong in the **Unknown**.

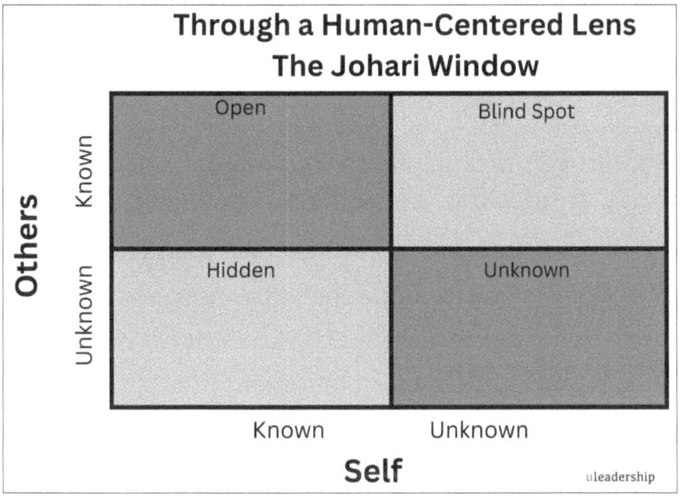

Step 4: Reflect

- What surprised you?
- Which traits would you like to move into the **Open Self** by sharing more of yourself?
- How can you reduce your **Blind Spots** by seeking constructive feedback?

Note: The Human-Centered Johari Window is based on interpretations of work originally produced by Joseph Luft and Harrington Ingham. You can read more in Joe Luft's 1969 book: *Of Human Interaction: Johari Model.*

Balancing internal and external self-awareness mirrors the gardener's work of fostering harmony between soil, plants, and the environment. Together, these dimensions create clarity, authenticity, and empathy, essential for personal growth and effective leadership. A flourishing garden captivates and uplifts all who behold it, much like a self-aware leader with a strong sense of well-being. Their positive influence radiates outward, enriching the lives they touch and transforming the environments they navigate.

Just as self-awareness forms the foundation of HCL, the ability to manage our emotions and reactions—known as self-regulation or emotional intelligence—builds on this foundation. Self-regulation is the conscious choice to control and redirect emotions, allowing us to pause and reflect before acting. This practice helps leaders experience emotions fully without being overwhelmed, fostering integrity, trustworthiness, and adaptability.

Leaders who can name their emotions stay calm under pressure, remain focused on their goals, and inspire trust and confidence in their teams. Yet, even the most poised leaders can struggle with emotional control when under extreme stress. I once worked with a nurse manager who was known for her calm demeanor and steady leadership, even in chaotic situations. However, one particularly overwhelming day brought an influx of patient admissions, supply shortages, and low staffing. Frustrated and overwhelmed, she lost her temper and lashed out at her colleagues. This outburst fractured the team's confidence and communication, creating tension that lingered for days.

Recognizing the damage, the nurse manager took intentional steps to rebuild trust and repair the harm caused by her actions. She apologized sincerely, sought stress management training, and introduced regular support meetings for staff. Over time, the team healed, becoming stronger and more resilient. This experience underscored the importance of emotional control and the profound impact a leader's behavior can have on their team.

However, maintaining emotional balance requires more than just self-control—it calls for self-compassion. When leaders make mistakes, as all humans do, reflecting with kindness and understanding allows them to learn and grow without being consumed by self-criticism. Showing ourselves compassion can be challenging, especially in a culture that often equates success with perfection. As Brené Brown (2010) explains in her bestselling book, *The Gifts of Imperfection*, striving for perfection isn't about becoming our best selves—it's a "20-ton shield" used to protect against vulnerability. This shield may prevent judgment or shame but often leads to anxiety, fear of failure, and stifled growth. Instead, practicing self-compassion—recognizing our shared humanity, embracing imperfection, and extending kindness to ourselves—cultivates fortitude and supports a growth mindset. It allows us to recover from setbacks, navigate challenges, and become the best versions of ourselves.

Leadership, much like gardening, is an ongoing practice of nurturing ourselves and others. At its foundation lies self-awareness, the ability to understand our emotions, values, and actions, which shapes how we show up in the world. Building on this foundation is self-regulation—the conscious choice to manage and redirect emotions—fostering integrity, adaptability, and trustworthiness. Paired with self-compassion, these practices help leaders recover from setbacks, embrace imperfections, and nurture a growth mindset. The authentic leader embodies all these qualities, allowing their true self to shine through their actions, decisions, and words. Authenticity is the heart of HCL. It means understanding who you are at your core—your strengths, limitations, beliefs, and passions—and letting this self-awareness guide how you interact with others and make choices.

Final Thoughts on Becoming a Master Gardener!

Being authentic as a leader is about transparency, integrity, and vulnerability. It's about admitting when you don't have all the answers and making decisions rooted not just in strategy but in empathy and ethical responsibility. When leaders lead with authenticity, they foster an environment of trust and care, inspiring those they lead to show up as their true selves.

Authenticity is deeply intertwined with well-being. When you are true to yourself, you experience fewer internal conflicts and less self-doubt. Effective leaders align their actions and decisions with their values, boosting self-esteem and cultivating a sense of fulfillment. Authentic leaders also communicate transparently, fostering trust and credibility within their teams, and show empathy and compassion toward their colleagues, ensuring their well-being is a priority.

Moreover, authenticity creates fortitude—an ability to navigate setbacks with grace and maintain a positive, forward-thinking attitude. This fortitude enables leaders to inspire their teams with a compelling vision for the future, even during challenging times. By being true to themselves, authentic leaders serve as role models, empowering those around them to thrive and embrace their individuality.

Just as tending a garden requires care and attention to every detail—from the soil to the weeds—HCL calls for intentionality and dedication to the self. Through authenticity, leaders cultivate trust, connection, and growth within their teams and communities. Ultimately, the authenticity of a leader not only shapes their well-being but also inspires positive change and fortitude in those they lead. Remember, it starts with you!

Discussion Questions for Groups

1. Why is authenticity important in both personal well-being and leadership? How can embracing vulnerability and being true to yourself influence trust and connection within a team or community?
2. Reflecting on the story of the nurse manager, how can self-regulation and emotional intelligence shape team dynamics and outcomes in high-pressure

situations? How do you personally manage your emotions when facing challenges?

3. What practices or habits do you use to maintain a sense of well-being, and how do they influence your ability to lead or support others? How can leaders encourage well-being within their teams or organizations?

Reflection Questions for Individuals

1. Brené Brown describes perfectionism as a "shield" that can hinder personal growth and connection. How have you experienced the impact of perfectionism in your own life or work, and what steps have you taken (or can you take) to cultivate self-compassion and a growth mindset?

   ____

   ____

   ____

   ____

   ____

2. Use the Wheel of Well-Being and list of guided questions and take time to debrief with yourself. Take time with each question, journaling your thoughts or discussing them with a trusted friend or mentor. Once you've identified areas for growth, celebrate your strengths and set small, achievable goals for improvement in dimensions where you feel less balanced.

   ____

   ____

   ____

   ____

   ____

References

Brown, B. (2010). *The gifts of imperfection: Let go of who you think you're supposed to be and embrace who you are.* Hazelden Publishing.

Kennedy, K., Leclerc, L., & Campis, S. (2022). *Human-centered leadership in healthcare: Evolution of a revolution.* Morgan James.

Luft, J. (1969). *Of human interaction.* National Press Books.

Recommended Reading

Beck, M. (2021). *The way to integrity: Finding the path to your true self.* Penguin Random House.

Brown, B. (2010). *The gifts of imperfection: Let go of who you think you're supposed to be and embrace who you are.* Hazelden Publishing.

Lowes, R. (2020). Knowing you: Personal tutoring, learning analytics, and the Johari Window. *Frontiers in Education, 5*, Article 101.

Oliver, S., & Duncan, S. (2019). Editorial: Looking through the Johari window. *Research for All, 3*(1): 1–6. doi: 10.18546/RFA.03.1.01

CHAPTER 5

The Language— "I Matter"

You might be but one drop in a bigger ocean, but even that drop causes ripples that affect every other drop.

—Sue Krebs, Author and Spiritual Teacher

The Essence of Mattering: Beyond Visibility

What does it mean to matter? Most people instinctively equate it with visibility—with being seen, heard, or acknowledged. Maybe having your post go viral, or receiving applause after delivering a speech, or better yet, having lots of people attend your birthday party are moments that feel like proof of significance, confirmation that we exist in a way that holds weight. But is recognition the measure of mattering? If no one sees us, do we cease to have value?

Perhaps mattering is less about attention and more about impact. A quiet act of kindness, a lesson passed down from generation to generation, a decision that shifts the course of someone's life—these might never make headlines, but they shape the world in ways that can't be measured by likes or recognition. Consider figures such as Rosalind Franklin, whose groundbreaking work in X-ray crystallography laid the foundation for the discovery of DNA's structure, or Katherine Johnson, whose mathematical brilliance ensured the success of early NASA missions—both women worked behind the scenes, shaping the future in ways the world took decades to fully acknowledge (Isaacson, 2021; Shetterly, 2016). Some of the most influential figures in history worked in the shadows, never knowing the full effect of their contributions. Does that make them any less significant? Or does it remind us that true significance isn't measured by visibility, but by the lasting impact we leave on others—whether or not we ever see it unfold?

So, why does "mattering" matter in leadership? According to Ellington (2023), mattering influences many aspects of leadership including employee engagement, motivation, job satisfaction, and overall organizational performance. The concept of "mattering" naturally complements the key attributes of Human-Centered Leadership (HCL): self-awareness, self-compassion, and mindfulness (Table 1). These aren't just trendy buzzwords or trends—they're essential practices that help us understand ourselves and our place within the universe. Each one acts like a compass, guiding us toward a stronger sense of identity and purpose. When we feel like we matter, we begin to see the significance of our existence—not only for ourselves but also for the people and the world around us. Mattering isn't dependent on validation—it manifests in the spaces between recognition. It lives in the ripple effect of the choices we make, the values we uphold, and the relationships we nurture. Often, we don't get to witness the full impact of our words, actions, or presence, but that doesn't make them any less significant. So perhaps the real question isn't "Do I matter?" because we know we do, but rather "Where does my mattering show up, even when I don't see it?"

TABLE 1 Defined Attributes of Human-Centered Leadership in Healthcare: Self

Self	Practices to support self
Well-Being	Approaches life satisfaction through a holistic, subjective, and multidimensional approach while finding balance in the elements of physical, emotional, social, spiritual, intellectual, and financial health.
Self-Care	Maintains a healthy relationship with self, focusing on physical, mental, and spiritual care. The way we treat ourselves.
Self-Compassion	Views life struggles with understanding, kindness, and grace. The way we relate to ourselves.
Self-Aware	Understands the underlying intentions that steer our thoughts, actions, and behaviors. The way we see ourselves.
Mindfulness	Checks in with self in the moment to note and acknowledge feelings and thoughts.

Note: Adapted from Leclerc, Kennedy, and Campis (2021).

Mattering and Human-Centered Leadership : Feeling Valued

In their book *How People Matter: Why It Affects Health, Happiness, Love, Work, and Society*, Isaac Prilleltensky and Ora Prilleltensky (2021) explore a simple yet profound truth about being human: We all want to feel valued and to know that we're contributing something meaningful to the world. It's a universal need, yet it holds the power to shape how we view ourselves and how we connect with others.

Self-awareness is a powerful and enlightening tool that invites us to truly understand ourselves. It involves examining our strengths, values, thoughts, and behaviors to uncover the essence of who we are. While we often think of self-awareness as asking life's profound questions—Who am I? What do I care about? What makes me unique?—it also encompasses the everyday, moment-to-moment reflections.

What am I feeling right now? What is my intention in this situation? Does my behavior align with my values and goals? And if not, why? By taking intentional pauses to acknowledge our emotions, clarify our intentions, and identify our strengths, we start to see how these elements shape the way we perceive the world, make decisions, and contribute to our surroundings.

This practice empowers us to celebrate our individuality and embrace the unique qualities that define us. Self-awareness not only fosters personal growth but also reminds us that we are creators of our own experiences—actively shaping the world through our authenticity and purpose.

This realization nurtures a sense of purpose and value, reminding us that we are not merely participants in life; we are active architects of our experiences. Feeling valued starts with appreciating what makes us unique.

At the same time, self-awareness allows us to appreciate the diversity of minds around us. Each person sees the world through a different lens, shaped by their experiences, values, and ways of thinking. Comparing minds isn't about measuring one's worth against another—it's about recognizing how different perspectives complement each other, how they challenge assumptions, and how they spark new ideas.

It's easy to fall into the comparison trap, thinking our contributions pale in comparison to others. But the truth is, the world thrives on diversity. Our unique quirks, passions, and perspectives enrich relationships, communities, and society as a whole. When we embrace the differences in how we think, we create environments that foster innovation, empathy, and collective growth.

Instead of seeing comparisons as competition, we can see them as an opportunity to learn. The beauty of HCL lies in its ability to highlight the value in every individual voice—not by diminishing differences, but by celebrating them. Our value, however, is not just a reflection of how we see ourselves; it often emerges most clearly in how we connect with others. When we feel truly valued, it's often because someone has recognized our worth, celebrated our contributions, and encouraged us to share our unique perspectives. This reciprocal exchange—valuing and being valued—fosters stronger, more authentic relationships. It reminds us that our individuality is not a barrier, but a bridge, connecting us with those around us.

The concept of embracing uniqueness extends beyond personal relationships and into the broader contexts of work, communities, and society. In professional environments, for example, recognizing the diverse talents and viewpoints of team members can transform collaboration. It allows people to bring their authentic selves to the table, fueling creativity and innovation. When leaders model this by creating spaces where every voice is heard and respected, they foster an atmosphere where both individuals and the collective can thrive.

Embracing diversity isn't limited to what makes us different—it's also about finding common threads. Amid our varying strengths, passions, and quirks, there is a shared humanity that connects us all. This awareness makes us more compassionate, more open to understanding, and more willing to grow together.

As we celebrate our own and others' uniqueness, we begin to see comparison in a new light—not as a measure of "better" or "worse," but as an opportunity to expand our horizons. Each mind, with its unique way of seeing the world, offers a piece of the puzzle. Together, these pieces form a richer, more intricate picture—one that no single perspective could create on its own.

Mattering and HCL: Adding Value

Adding value means channeling those strengths into meaningful actions. Perhaps you're a creative thinker who spots opportunities others miss. Or maybe you're the calming presence during a crisis, offering clarity and reassurance. Whatever your strengths, they're tools for making an impact—whether by helping one person, solving a problem, or advancing a cause that's close to your heart. When each of us feels safe and encouraged to recognize and share our strengths, a culture of significance takes shape (Mercurio, 2025).

Identifying and embracing our strengths helps us honor our individuality and recognize what we bring to the table. Speaking of what we bring to the table, have you ever been to a potluck? A good potluck is all about variety—everyone shows up with something delicious yet unique. Imagine a potluck where everyone brought fried chicken. Now, I love fried chicken as much as anyone, but no one wants a meal that's entirely the same. You need potato salad, corn on the cob, fresh tomatoes, juicy watermelon—now that's a meal worth remembering! The magic of a potluck is in the mix—different dishes coming together to create something special.

In many ways, a potluck is a great metaphor for our unique strengths. Every person brings their own "dish" to life's table—a blend of talents, perspectives, and experiences that no one else can replicate. These qualities not only shape who we are but also remind us that we're valuable and capable of making a difference. Embracing what makes us distinct is like showing up to the potluck with our best dish, ready to enrich the feast of life. It's empowering to see ourselves not just as participants in life, but as creators and contributors. That realization is what helps us feel truly valued. By celebrating our strengths and integrating them into our self-awareness, we unlock the potential to make meaningful contributions and inspire others along the way. It's a continuous process that reinforces our sense of worth and helps us navigate life with clarity, confidence, and authenticity.

Self-compassion builds on this foundation, teaching us to treat ourselves with kindness and grace, even during moments of doubt or failure. It's about recognizing that being imperfect doesn't lessen our worth. When we practice self-compassion, we become less critical and more accepting of ourselves, creating space for growth and resilience. This self-acceptance gives us the confidence to pursue what matters most to us.

Then, there's mindfulness, which grounds us in the present moment. In today's fast-paced world, mindfulness invites us to slow down and focus on what truly matters. It helps us align our actions with our values and create meaningful contributions, no matter how small. Whether it's offering a kind word, lending a helping hand, or taking time to reflect, mindfulness shows us that every moment holds the potential for significance.

Feeling like we matter isn't about grand gestures or monumental achievements. More often, it's found in quiet, everyday actions and positive habits. It's about pausing to recognize the value of our contributions, no matter how insignificant they might seem. A simple act of kindness, a listening ear, or a steady presence can ripple outward, creating impacts we may never fully realize. Recognizing and understanding our emotions is essential, as they hold significant power in shaping our experiences—whether toward a positive or negative perspective. Developing this awareness allows us to navigate our emotions more effectively and influence the outcomes of our experiences in meaningful ways. When we first acknowledge our value, we're better equipped to create value for others and society, fostering greater satisfaction, happiness, and overall well-being in the process.

Connecting to the Bigger Picture

At its core, mattering connects us to a larger story. It's not just about self-worth—it's about seeing ourselves as part of a greater tapestry of people, ideas, and actions. When we embrace self-awareness, self-compassion, and mindfulness, we're not just discovering who we are; we're uncovering the countless ways we contribute to a better world simply by being ourselves.

The concept of mattering bridges these practices. When we take pride in our abilities and see how they contribute to something larger, we're reminded that we're part of a bigger picture. Whether your strength lies in kindness, innovation, humility, or leadership, it's not just about the ability itself—it's about how it connects you to others and helps build something greater.

So, take a moment to reflect: What are your unique strengths? How do they help you feel valued, and how do they enable you to add value to the world around you? When you embrace what makes you unique, you're not just meeting a need—you're living out the beautiful truth that you matter.

Understanding that you matter and have value softens your internal dialogue. Self-compassion helps you forgive your mistakes and appreciate your efforts, creating a more nurturing inner world. Mindfulness complements this by grounding you in the present, enhancing your sense of purpose and intention. Together, they form a foundation that reminds you that your actions ripple outward, touching lives in meaningful ways.

At its core, mattering transcends self-esteem—it encompasses purpose, connection, and the understanding that even the smallest actions can carry immense significance. For a leader in healthcare, recognizing our own value, adopting the philosophy of "It Starts With Me," and prioritizing our well-being, form the foundation of success as an Awakener, Connector, and Upholder. This perspective not only guides our personal growth but also enhances our ability to inspire and empower others. It's a beautiful way to approach life, wouldn't you agree?

Discussion Questions for Groups

1. What does "mattering" mean to you personally, and how does it influence the way you view your role in relationships, community, and society as a whole?

2. How can practices such as self-awareness, self-compassion, and mindfulness help us better recognize and embrace our unique strengths? Can you share examples from your own life?
3. In what ways do our individual strengths contribute to the "potluck" of life? How can we celebrate and make space for the diverse talents and perspectives of others?
4. Why is it sometimes challenging to see our own value or feel that we matter? How can we overcome these challenges and support others in feeling valued as well?

Reflection Questions for Individuals

Creating positive emotions starts with a mindset of gratitude. Consider ways to nurture a mindset of gratitude. Here are some ideas to get you started.

1. **Gratitude Journaling**:
   - What are three things I am grateful for today, and why?
   - How does expressing gratitude shift my mindset and emotions?

   ____

   ____

   ____

   ____

   ____

2. **Acknowledging Kindness**:
   - Who has positively impacted my life recently? How can I express appreciation in a meaningful way?
   - What does receiving gratitude feel like, and how does it reinforce my sense of self-worth?

   ____

   ____

   ____

   ____

   ____

3. **Embracing the Present**:
   - What past worries or regrets am I holding onto, and how can I gently release them?
   - In this very moment, what simple joys or blessings can I fully embrace?

   ____

   ____

   ____

   ____

   ____

References

Ellington, L. M. (2023). Mattering: Shaping organizational leadership practices. *Journal of Leadership Studies, 17*(2), 45–58.

Isaacson, W. (2021). *The code breaker: Jennifer Doudna, gene editing, and the future of the human race.* Simon & Schuster.

Leclerc, L., Kennedy, K., & Campis, S. (2021). Human-centred leadership in healthcare: A contemporary nursing leadership theory generated via constructivist grounded theory. *Journal of Nursing Management, 29*(2), 294–306.

Mercurio, Z. (2025). *The power of mattering: How leaders can create a culture of significance.* HarperCollins.

Prilleltensky, I., & Prilleltensky, O. (2021). *How people matter: Why it affects health, happiness, love, work, and society.* Cambridge University Press.

Shetterly, M. L. (2016). *Hidden figures: The American dream and the untold story of the Black women mathematicians who helped win the space race.* William Morrow.

Recommended Reading

Flett, G. L. (2018). *The psychology of mattering: Understanding the human need to be significant.* Academic Press.

Robinson, B. (2022). "Mattering" is the top leadership skill for retaining employees. *Forbes.*

PART III

But It's Not About You

Human-Centered Leadership in Healthcare (HCL-HC) begins with Self but finds its true impact in how leaders then focus their energy outward, on others. The Awakener, Connector, and Upholder shape environments where people flourish. This section presents research-backed updates to these leadership dimensions, refining their associated mindset and language for greater clarity and impact. Be sure to bookmark the chapter on stories from the field, *Real People, Real Results!*, which showcases how HCL-HC has been operationalized in real-world healthcare settings and produced real-world outcomes. Learn how HCL creates the conditions for collective success.

CHAPTER 6

But It's Not About You!

Leadership is not about control. Leadership is about influence.

—Ford Taylor, Author, leadership solutions trainer

Have you noticed the number of personality tests seems to be expanding? I first found out that I'm an ENFJ on the Myers-Briggs personality assessment (Myers-Briggs, n.d.); then, I learned I'm a collaborator and creator on the Competing Values Framework Model (Cameron & Quinn, n.d.). I'm an "I" on the DISC Personality Assessment Tool (Harris & Eikenberry, 2020), and I recently learned I'm an Enneagram Type 2 with a Type 3 Wing (Truity, 2020). So . . . who am I?

When it comes to Human-Centered Leadership in Healthcare (HCL-HC), rest assured you won't be categorized as simply an Awakener, a Connector, or an Upholder. Sure, you'll recognize yourself in the model and will most likely identify with one of these dimensions more so than the others. That simply means that you have insight into your leadership strengths, and you recognize the areas in which you have opportunities to grow. These relational leadership dimensions are interconnected and together create the culture change in healthcare that results in sustained outcomes. It's similar to the idea of well-being. To have a balanced and healthy life, you must focus on mind, body, and spirit since well-being in all three is necessary. The same is true for a human-centered leader. It's through the development of each dimension of others-focused leadership—the Awakener, the Connector, and the Upholder—that you create and sustain a healthy culture. If the only required outcomes in healthcare were patient experience and staff satisfaction, then perhaps you could focus primarily on the attributes of the Upholder. But what about the required outcomes of quality care, patient safety, team collaboration, staff engagement, population health, connection with the community—the list goes on. Obviously, the organization would not be able to survive, much less thrive, without a focus on all the many metrics that indicate value to the patient, the staff, the community, and the payors. It takes recognition of all the dimensions of Human-Centered Leadership (HCL) to achieve these results in our interconnected, complex world of healthcare.

When you take the self-assessment for HCL-HC (www.uleadership.com/assessment/), you may learn that you have a natural tendency toward the outward-facing dimension of the Awakener, for example, but need to develop the attributes of the Connector and the Upholder. As you learn more about the attributes, and about yourself, the strategies will guide you to build your ability to embody all three.

> Personal well-being, at a minimum, requires a balance of mind, body, and spirit. Similarly, the human-centered leader requires a balance of the attributes of the outward-facing dimensions: the Awakener, the Connector, and the Upholder.

In the story below, you'll see how a human-centered leader exemplifies the attributes of the Awakener, the Connector, and the Upholder. Because of the inherent complexity in healthcare, the interconnected dimensions of leadership produce a culture reflective of well-being in healthcare.

Exemplar: A Human-Centered Leader's Approach to Problem-Solving

A surgical unit noticed a slight uptick in the number of patient falls over three months. During the unit's daily safety huddle, the nurse manager, Jamal, suggested that the team investigate the cause of the increase and worked with the charge nurse to develop a unit-specific audit tool. Each day, the charge nurse assigned a staff nurse to perform the audit, and that nurse reported results during the safety huddle. The team posted the data daily and identified areas for improvement. They then presented the safety issue to the nursing professional governance council. During this meeting, a "falls champion" was identified for each shift. The falls champions met with Jamal to review the current audit tool, identify additional contributing factors, and begin a more thorough investigation of patient falls. Over the next several weeks, the falls champions, along with the charge nurse and Jamal, performed audits on every patient to determine if fall risk protocols were consistently in place for high-risk patients. The audits also included checking each patient bed to ensure the bed alarms were functioning properly. With daily reports at each safety huddle, the topic of patient falls became a shift-to-shift discussion among the team members. A team goal included 100% compliance with the high-risk fall protocol; however, during the audits, the team discovered issues with nonfunctioning bed alarms. Jamal arranged for the engineering team to meet with the falls champions, and together, they reviewed the audit of the beds and the bed alarm system. They noted that many bed alarm cords were unplugged from the wall because the small prongs inside the plugs had broken. The engineering team took inventory and replaced all broken cords. The falls champions began to reeducate the nursing team on the bed alarm system. The nurses identified the patient transport team as a group also requiring reeducation. Jamal worked with the falls champions to schedule educational sessions for the patient transport team. Continued audits for one month after the education sessions revealed no reported patient falls or near misses. The falls champions continued to audit and educate as needed. Over the next six-month period, there were no patient falls. Jamal planned a celebration for the unit to acknowledge their hard work and their successful result on this patient safety issue. Jamal also suggested that the falls champions submit their work as a best practice poster presentation at a local nursing conference. He reached out to the unit educator to serve as a mentor and coach for the two nurses who had served as falls champions. The nurses submitted their poster and were awarded second place for an innovative best practice.

Embodying an *Awakener:* Motivator, Mentor, Coach, Architect, and Advocate

Jamal recognized the problem with patient falls and quickly went to work engaging and *mentoring* the team. He believed in the wisdom and ability of the team and looked for ways to reveal excellence. His initial step, working with the charge nurse to develop an audit tool, exemplified the importance of including the leaders and nurses closest to the point of care to develop the solutions. The audit, performed by a unit nurse, was shared each day at the safety huddle, allowing the care team to own the data and use it as the basis for their learning. This real-time feedback enhanced the staff's connection to their purpose—to deliver high-quality and safe patient care (*motivator*).

The responsibility for the solution was handed off to the Professional Governance Council, the structure Jamal had built on the unit for point-of-care decision-making (*architect*). Also, a falls champion for each shift was elected, further enlarging the influence of the team. Jamal worked with the falls champions to tweak the audit tool based on their new knowledge and provided coaching on the improvement process.

Jamal advocated for the team by engaging the engineering department to work with the falls champions and remedy the technical problem related to the bed alarms. This problem with the bed alarms would likely not have been uncovered had Jamal gone about the process improvement in a different way. Imagine if instead, he had blamed the staff for being inattentive to their patients and being careless about using bed alarms. The staff would have possibly become disengaged and silent, and the engineering department would not have known a problem existed.

Lastly, Jamal recognized the staff for the solution by celebrating their success. He cleared the path for them to move forward with a poster presentation and ensured further mentoring and coaching by the unit educator. His actions contributed to the culture of excellence because he was comfortable being the Awakener, rather than the hero!

Embodying a *Connector:* Collaborator, Supporter, Edgewalker, Engineer, Authentic Communicator

Jamal understood that as a Connector, he didn't have to have all the answers. His main goal was to unify the team around the unit goals and trust them as the experts. He demonstrated *authentic communication* with the team as he gathered them for the safety huddle each day. He used open, honest communication to demonstrate his trust and respect for the team.

When the uptick in patient falls was noted, Jamal didn't overreact to the data by quickly putting a new initiative in place for the team to follow. A traditional leader might have instituted a falls checklist to be used by every nurse with every patient interaction and then monitored the team for compliance. Instead, Jamal embraced the problem as an opportunity for the team to innovate and problem-solve. By recognizing that problems are inevitable and embracing uncertainty as an opportunity for innovation, Jamal demonstrated the fine art of *edgewalking*. He knew how to hold the precise tension between essential processes while also being open to new learning, surprises, and innovation.

Jamal supported the findings of the Professional Governance Council and welcomed the opportunity for the staff to collaborate with the transport team on a shared goal. He knew that by engaging the falls champions in the process and using the skill of the unit educator, the solution would likely be more sustainable (*engineer*). Jamal's leadership behaviors contributed to a culture of trust because he trusted the wisdom of the team and connected both people and processes to develop a solution.

Embodying an *Upholder:* Personally Well, Mindful, Others-Oriented, Emotionally Aware, and Socially and Organizationally Aware

Jamal exemplified HCL by first recognizing that he didn't have all the answers. He was vulnerable with the team, recognizing them as the influencers and problem-solvers (*others-oriented*). He could have piled this responsibility on top of his already busy schedule and possibly overreacted due to the additional stress. Instead, he remained calm and present, likely able to attend to his own self-care (*personally well*). Through emotional awareness and mindfulness, he embedded himself within the team and demonstrated his trust and belief in their good intentions. There was no mention of blame or shame. Jamal's actions demonstrated he was concerned about the patients on the unit, rather than the uptick in the data and the reflection the data could have on him as the leader (others-oriented).

Lastly, Jamal was *socially* and *organizationally aware*. He knew how to collaborate with others outside the unit, e.g., the engineering department and the patient transporters, without placing blame. He demonstrated his ability to navigate organizational politics and bring people together around a shared purpose. By demonstrating the attributes of the Upholder, Jamal contributed to a culture of caring that impacted the satisfaction of both the caregivers and their patients.

This story illustrates how the four dimensions of the human-centered leader—Self, Awakener, Connector, and Upholder—are all interconnected. Together, they create a powerful synergy that influences not just the leader, but also the team, the broader interdisciplinary group, and ultimately, the patients. It's a perfect example of Aristotle's timeless wisdom: "The whole is greater than the sum of its parts." The real magic lies in the dynamic interactions, collaboration, and collective growth that these dimensions make possible.

Like any complex system, understanding the whole starts by breaking it down into its individual parts. That's exactly what we'll do in the next three chapters. We'll explore the three outward-facing dimensions of the human-centered leader—Awakener, Connector, and Upholder. You'll get practical insights on how to embrace these dimensions, bring their attributes to life, and integrate them seamlessly into your leadership style. Using the "Being, Knowing, and Doing" framework, we'll dive into how small, meaningful changes can spark personal and professional transformation. By the end, you'll see the truth in the statement: "It starts with you, but it's not about you."

Discussion Questions for Groups

1. As a leader, you have likely encountered an increase in a "never" event. How did you handle it? Does Jamal's story highlight any areas of leadership you could consider including?
2. Do you have a strong Professional Governance Council in place to refer a patient care problem, such as an increase in "never" events? If not, what are your next steps in developing this structure?
3. Have you considered using a team huddle to engage staff in problem-solving?
4. Consider the best practices provided in the exemplar. How can you share best practices across your organization and still maintain staff ownership?

Reflection Questions for Individuals

Think about the current culture of your unit or department. Does the culture reflect excellence, trust, and caring? Which area needs your attention and why?

____

____

____

____

____

References

Cameron, K., & Quinn, R. (n.d.). *The competing values culture assessment.* Competing Values Product Line. Retrieved from https://www.boomhogeronderwijs.nl/media/8/download_pdf_culture_assessment_workbook.pdf

Harris, G., & Eikenberry, K. (2020). *DISC personality test.* DISC Personality Testing. Retrieved from https://discpersonalitytesting.com/free-disc-test

The Myers-Briggs Company. (n.d.) *Myers-Briggs type indicator.* Retrieved from https://www.themyersbriggs.com/en-US/Products-and-Services/Myers-Briggs

Truity. (2020). *Enneagram Personality Test.* Retrieved from https://www.truity.com/test/enneagram-personality-test

Recommended Reading

Gregory, M. E., Lazzara, E. H., & Blickensderfer, E. (2024). Leadership in health care: What are some novel insights? *Psychology of Leaders and Leadership, 27*(1), 1–5.

Kennedy, K., Campis, S., & Leclerc, L. (2020). Human-centered leadership in healthcare: Creating change from the inside out. *Nurse Leader, 18*(3), 227–231.

Spanos, S., Leask, E., Patel, R., Datyner, M., Loh, E., & Braithwaite, J. (2024). Healthcare leaders navigating complexity: A scoping review of key trends in future roles and competencies. *BMC Medical Education, 24*, Article 720.

CHAPTER 7

The Awakener

Developing a Culture of Excellence

I am not a teacher but an awakener.

—Robert Frost, American poet

There are those leaders, in academia or in practice, who are particularly strong in the attributes of the Awakener primarily because of their natural gift in education and professional development. I want to share a story about a clinical nurse specialist who definitively embodies the attributes of the Awakener as a way of highlighting and examining each attribute more closely. I hope this story causes you to think about leaders in your journey who knew how to recognize potential and reveal the excellence that already existed within each team member.

From Passion to Practice: Awakening Excellence in Critical Care

As the leader of critical care services, I had the honor of working with a clinical nurse specialist, Barbara McLean, a renowned expert in critical care. She was passionate about sharing her knowledge of critical care nursing with bedside staff in a way that made the science of caring for the critically ill come to life. The nurses entrusted to Barbara's teaching felt honored and "special" to be her mentees and wore that sense of belonging and accomplishment as a badge. Barbara held a high bar for participation in education and established a culture where expertise was expected, authentic care for the patient was essential, and continued growth strengthened the nurses' purpose and belonging. Her passion for excellence overflowed in each interaction and she exemplified the saying that "knowledge is power." Despite her "power," she demonstrated the utmost humility and respect for everyone on the team.

Barbara developed the orientation program to prepare surgical/trauma intensive care nurses to advance their learning and become the expert staff needed to care for patients undergoing cardiac surgery. This was a new program added at a large public hospital to complete the cardiac service line. The orientation program was rigorous and included learning to read EKG strips, recognize ST-elevation myocardial infarctions, provide acute and post-acute care of ST-elevation myocardial infarctions patients, and provide post-op care to cardiac surgery patients. The nurses who took on this additional workload and training were internally motivated by the desire to become better and, frankly, to become more like Barbara. Since Barbara had established herself as an expert in critical care, she modeled the expertise and leadership that the best of the best intensive care unit (ICU) nurses wanted to emulate.

The nurses in this program owned their development and worked as a team to provide the support needed for the overall program. In the early stages of the program, they mapped out a schedule to be sure at least one of them was slated to work in the ICU each shift. They did this to ensure the level of care for cardiac patients would be optimal, should a patient require it. The other nurses on the unit, who were not a part of the advanced cohort, equally shared in the collaboration as they supported their "cardiac" teammates.

The cardiac cohort of nurses spent hours in the classroom, studied and reviewed EKGs, and took comprehension and applicability tests. Because of their personal investment, they owned their outcomes and were committed to the success of the program. Along with their commitment came the confidence and empowerment to freely bring forward concerns and disagreements with surgeons and other members of the healthcare team if it meant they could together improve trust and communication. The authentic communication and productive conflict around different perspectives pushed the team to become better and contributed to the program's huge success.

As a result of their ownership of the program and their desire to make it as comprehensive as possible, the team self-organized, with Barbara's oversight, into a chest pain evaluation team. They wanted to be sure that inpatients who had symptoms of cardiac ischemia had access to the same rapid diagnosis and treatment as patients admitted through the emergency department. The rapid response team, traditionally the team that responds to patients in cardiac arrest, was educated on the process and began responding to in-house episodes of chest pain. The nurses were successful as first responders in their assessment of patients, collaboration with the cardiologists, and ability to move the patient through the algorithm for prompt diagnosis and treatment. Barbara was, of course, right there with them—one of the team.

As the program progressed, one of the surgeons had the idea of standardizing the handoff at the bedside from cardiac surgery to critical care. The cardiac nurses took the lead and established the handoff process from the cardiac surgery operating room team to the critical care team of physicians, nurses, and other disciplines. When a patient arrived in the ICU after cardiac surgery, the interprofessional team gathered at the bedside for a thorough handoff on the patient's care. As you may have guessed, the cardiac nurses led the handoff and ensured that the prescribed process was consistently followed.

Leaders like Barbara, *natural* Awakeners, stir the excellence that already exists in their team. Barbara's leadership ignited the team's desire to grow because she modeled continuous learning, invested in each staff member, set a high bar for engagement, and created a learning environment. Barbara and the nurses celebrated every learning milestone and patient success, which, along with their sense of self-accomplishment, provided the fuel needed to keep the team highly engaged.

While this story is about an exceptional clinical leader, all human-centered leaders, with differing levels of expertise, can model the characteristics of an Awakener. As an Awakener, you set the expectation for continuous learning and infuse it into clinical practice through collaboration with clinical experts. I mentioned that Barbara was an extremely humble leader who worked hard to keep her collaborative relationships strong. She credited the team with every success. An Awakener never takes on the attitude of the "hero" but instead elevates those on the team who have worked to deserve the respect associated with excellence.

Quality programs in healthcare typically refer to "loop closure" as a way to continuously study and improve processes related to patient care. This hospital accomplished loop closure for the cardiac service line by studying each case as a collaborative team. The team included emergency medical services, cardiologists, nursing leaders, a cardiac catheterization lab team member, and a quality expert. When at all possible, one of the staff nurses from the cardiac cohort attended as well. The team tried to learn from each case and then implemented changes based on their new knowledge. This is what true accountability looks like.

It's easy to see the impact of the Awakener through Barbara's story. Again, the purpose of this story is to help you better understand the attributes of an Awakener so you can work to develop them in your leadership practice. The payoff comes as your behaviors impact the staff, the patient, and the environment. To be effective, you don't need to become a world-renowned expert in your clinical area like Barbara, but you do need to set the expectations of growth and development and create a learning environment as you collaborate with clinical experts. When you embrace the attributes of the Awakener, you'll see that the team owns their individual and collaborative practice and implements innovative solutions based on their new knowledge (Leclerc, Kennedy, & Campis, 2020). In short, keep your sights on "awakening" excellence in each staff member. By embracing the attributes of the Awakener, your team will achieve market-leading outcomes, and the ultimate success will be realized by the patient who receives the highest quality care. If one of my family members requires cardiac care, I would not hesitate to take them to the hospital described here. I know, firsthand, that the nursing care there is *excellent*.

Start with Self: *Be* the Awakener

To become the kind of leader who unlocks potential in others—helping them grow, thrive, and surpass their own expectations—your values and mindset must be at the core. It begins with self-reflection: embracing vulnerability, committing to continuous growth, and embodying a purposeful career and meaningful life. Prioritize your well-being, recognizing that your life's satisfaction profoundly influences how you show up as a leader. Know your purpose, reflect on it daily, and challenge yourself to remain true to it. Model the value of continuous learning—your actions will set the bar and inspire others to follow. Be comfortable admitting when you don't have all the answers and own your mistakes with humility. Who you are at your core—the alignment of your values and mindset—shapes your intentions and is evident in your actions. If your goal is to inspire the growth and development of others, the journey must first begin with you.

Cultivating the Mindset of an Awakener: Seeking Excellence

The mindset of an Awakener begins with actively looking for excellence in others. Consider the experience of learning a new word and suddenly noticing it everywhere—in conversations, books, or media. Or considering purchasing a particular car, only to see it appear frequently on the highway. What you focus on is what you'll find. To spot excellence in your team, you must deliberately train your eye to seek it out. Identify strengths and voice them; look beyond what people can do now to envision their potential—and provide the nudge they need to reach it. Resist the urge to step in and fix problems. Instead, offer people the space to navigate challenges and discover their own solutions. Finally, embrace the long game—growth takes time, and patience is key.

As you deepen your understanding of the Awakener and transition from *being* to *knowing*, remember that your ultimate goal is to spark a desire within each team member to learn, grow, and reach beyond what they once thought possible. Achieving this requires a genuine interest in the individuals on your team and an unwavering belief in their untapped potential. Reflect on a moment in your own journey when a leader or teacher believed in you—pushing you to achieve more than you imagined. It's both humbling and empowering to receive such validation, creating a ripple effect that extends far beyond the moment. This type of relational leadership begins with your inward focus—embracing vulnerability, committing to continuous growth, and living a purposeful and meaningful life (Figure 4).

The Language of the Awakener—"I believe in you."

The Awakener harnesses the language, "I believe in you," as a profound catalyst for igniting motivation and unlocking potential. These words, paired with actions like celebrating achievements, offering mentorship, and encouraging autonomy, reflect genuine confidence in team members' capabilities. This affirmation inspires individuals to push beyond their comfort zones, enhancing their sense of purpose and ownership. Over time, this trust—expressed consistently in both words and actions—creates a culture of growth, resilience, and empowerment, fueling excellence within the team. Let's dive deeper into the attributes of the Awakener to explore how these powerful words—"I believe in you"—come to life.

Awaken Others Through *Knowing*

The attributes of the Awakener include motivator, mentor, coach, architect, and advocate (Table 2). As you learn more about these attributes in the sections below, pay attention to how real-world nurses and healthcare leaders bring them to life in practice. We cite some of the examples and quotes from our original research, which have been validated through ongoing inquiry over the past few years.

FIGURE 4
The Awakener.

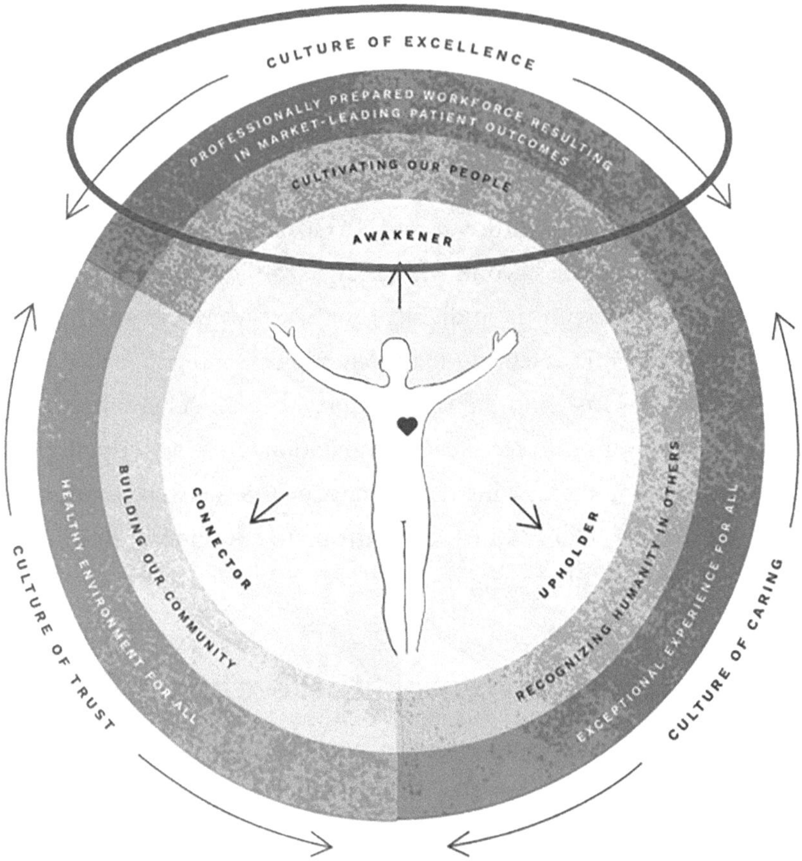

Note: Adapted from Leclerc, Kennedy, and Campis (2021).

TABLE 2	Defined Attributes Embodied by the Human-Centered Leader as an Awakener
Awakener	**Cultivates our people**
Motivator	Establishes a learning culture that leverages the power of the individual's intrinsic motivation.
Coach	Provides honest feedback addressing strengths and opportunities to improve performance.
Mentor	Advises on professional career path and actions to achieve goals.
Architect	Designs structures and processes so innovation can emerge.
Advocate	Ensures resources are available for best practice and professional growth.

Note: Adapted from Leclerc, Kennedy, and Campis (2021).

Motivator

As leaders, we know that you cannot force someone to become motivated. Motivation comes from within. You can, however, help connect personal and professional growth opportunities with the individual staff member's goals and sense of purpose. As you get to know each team member, seek to understand their goals and *look for opportunities* to connect them to their goals and purpose. This is a key step in awakening excellence within individuals.

You will learn that establishing a learning environment is motivating to your team. When problem-solving, there should be multidirectional dialogue with the staff rather than one-way communication from you to the staff. If you provide a definitive linear process to achieve a goal, the team has little ownership of the process or the results. You will find yourself monitoring the process and becoming frustrated with the team's lack of motivation to comply. If you instead develop a learning environment and allow the team to experiment, based on their experience and researched best practices, they will be motivated to develop processes that work for them and meet the desired outcomes. A learning environment connects the staff to their internal motivation to grow professionally and provide the best care for their patients.

As you focus on learning, don't hesitate to hold a high, but reachable, bar for continued growth. Clearly communicate that the high bar stems from a passionate desire to provide the utmost expertise and the highest quality of care for patients. Setting the high bar also reflects your belief in the team's capabilities. Unless the bar is a stretch, requiring a significant investment, accomplishing the goals won't carry the same sense of pride that develops into a motivating passion. In Barbara's case, she had to remove nurses from the cohort if they didn't meet the rigorous expectations. There's no trophy for being a passive member of the team. Barbara required a substantial investment in the work, knowing this would gain the most valuable dividends for the team members (and the patients).

As your team members feel motivated and empowered by their learning, there is an infectious spread to others. Nurses own their professional growth to ensure their expertise and confidence in providing exceptional care to their patients. This provides a way for the nurses to connect to and sustain their purpose—making a difference in the lives of patients by providing high-quality patient care.

To further connect to staff members' internal motivation, encourage each member to develop an individual professional growth plan to help them stay connected to continued growth and purpose. This plan should be reviewed as a part of their annual employee performance appraisal. The employee owns their growth plan, and your role is to encourage, mentor, support, and advocate for each of them as they work through their plan. The nurses in our original research referred to this as *extending ownership for growth while offering support*. Those not interested in meeting the challenge to grow professionally will typically self-select out of the unit because their lack of engagement will set them apart from the team.

Motivator in Action: A new nurse begins work on a medical–surgical unit, and you learn from your conversation with him that his goal is to provide global nursing care to underserved populations through a nonprofit organization. He wants to learn as much as possible about medical–surgical nursing in preparation for an autonomous practice. Your role as a motivator is to tie his professional goals to those of the unit by seeking out opportunities that will build his knowledge, confidence, and expertise. You might also look for opportunities for him to be a member of a problem-solving team and eventually a team leader. Together, discuss what success will look like for him and what steps are needed to get there.

Mentor

As you develop the attributes of the Awakener, you'll recognize the value of becoming a mentor. The nurses in our original research felt that a mentor *promotes growth* for individuals and *builds the team.* As a mentor, you will become a model for others because you possess the required professional skills and even more importantly, you live your personal values. Our nurse participants listed *honesty, transparency, trust, communication, appropriate flexibility, self-development, and self-care* as valuable characteristics of a mentor. Mentors are in the business of developing other leaders, so as a mentor, you will interpret and model the characteristics and role of the leader to others.

As you mentor your staff, especially those new to their careers, you will expose them to different, challenging situations. If they are to build on important steps and missteps, you must allow room for learning and for inevitable errors. This will require foresight, flexibility, and patience. As a mentor, you need to clear the path to make these opportunities available at the right time to the right team members. As your relationship develops and you learn of specific behaviors they are trying to develop, the relationship can evolve into one-to-one coaching.

Mentor in Action: You are the manager of a medical–surgical unit, and a relatively new nurse on the unit lets you know that she would like to become a charge nurse. You know she's not ready yet, but as a mentor, you look for ways to expose her to different aspects of the position. You have her work with a seasoned charge nurse to develop competencies such as leading huddles, making assignments, and ensuring patient flow. Your organization has access to a leadership program to help develop new leaders, so you provide this opportunity as well. You also encourage other nurses working on the transition to become charge nurses to become peer coaches for each other. Over time, the staff nurse will learn and grow from her own mistakes and will learn where further coaching would help achieve her goal of becoming a charge nurse.

Coach

As you develop your skills as a coach, you'll recognize the significance of honest and thoughtful feedback to further each team member's growth. Often feedback is best received in the form of a question, born out of curiosity, which allows the nurse to discover the answer for themself. The intent of feedback is to improve practice and to reveal blind spots that may stem from years of habit or a lack of awareness. Through thoughtful and sensitive coaching, you will bring blind spots into the light, discuss opportunities for change, and look for progress rather than perfection. Through direct

Coach in Action: Consider the medical–surgical nurse in the previous story who wanted to become a charge nurse. As a mentor, you've ensured she was exposed to the tasks required of a charge nurse, participated in peer coaching, and completed a self-directed leadership course. She lets you know the area she needs to develop by assigning new admissions to team members. She states that she lacks confidence in her decisions. As a coach, ask about her biggest concern and what she thinks would give her more confidence in her ability to make sound decisions in this area. It may be that she needs practice walking through the process in real time. Discuss possible solutions such as working through the decision with other charge nurses or working through the decision with a peer coach. You don't always have to be the coach yourself, but you must ensure that the staff member receives the coaching they need to progress forward. Remember that everyone needs a coach; it's not a sign of weakness but a sign of initiative and motivation.

and honest feedback, you must acknowledge the humanity of each individual and establish an environment where team members can focus on specific areas for improvement. As a coach, you're conscious of not telling the team member what to do, which could be interpreted as micromanaging. Instead, you help the individual staff member determine appropriate next steps and encourage movement toward progress. Since the human-centered leader understands the work and the perspective of the staff members, the feedback, delivered sensitively, will likely be well received. As a coach, you will expect mistakes and setbacks. Use these as opportunities for further learning through the practice of reflection.

Architect

Let's go back for a moment to consider the earlier analogy of the downtown hospital under construction. As you grow in the attributes of the Awakener, you will function as an architect and will build the invisible infrastructure that supports the team's growth. The infrastructure includes core values that are lived every day such as respect, commitment to self, commitment to the team, and dedication to expertise in patient care (Tye & Dent, 2024). In addition, the infrastructure includes a Professional Governance Council, operational processes, and interconnections with multidisciplinary professionals. These components support the work of the team and the team's ability to achieve a culture of excellence.

The nurses in our research stated that their most admired leaders were able to develop and communicate a vision. They were able to *see a way forward and communicate to the team how to get there.* A vision co-created by the nurses and the leader contributes further to the infrastructure of the unit and has the fingerprints of the team all over it. As a human-centered leader, the plan for *how to get there* is developed *with* the team's input and ownership, so the leader is not the sole owner, but the team working together through supportive structures creates the vision for moving forward.

In today's complex environment, with ever-growing financial constraints, you will need to be creative and leverage resources to provide ample time for nurses to work together in problem-solving teams. Professional Governance may look different than it did in the past. Decision-making might need to take place during brief huddles rather than in separate meetings. Either way, decision-making at the point of care must continue to exist and evolve. The interconnectedness of the team within and outside the unit, supported by the invisible infrastructure, is the key to influencing positive change throughout the organization.

Architect in Action: As you consider the attributes of the architect, assess the current core values, decision-making structure, policies, and interconnections across the unit and hospital. Even though we refer to these as the *invisible* infrastructure, they should be very clear components to you and the team members. This infrastructure supports the way you do things on the unit and in the organization and incorporates the vision for achieving excellence. You may find it helpful to ask new team members about their perception of the infrastructure to be sure that you and the team are making the invisible visible.

Advocate

Lastly, our research confirmed that being an Awakener means serving as an advocate. As an advocate, you will act as a resource, and when necessary, connect team members with other knowledgeable individuals. According to one of the nurses from our research, *If they don't know the answer, they know where to go to find the answer.* As an advocate, you'll represent the team, and because of your position and being embedded in the work, you'll better understand the perspective of the team. By advocating for the team, it will be clear that your intention is to facilitate an environment that breeds empowerment among the nurses.

The tools and ability to research best practices around point-of-care concerns are resources your team will need. They will also need to know how to adjust best practices to fit the organization. This will be your opportunity to ensure there are members on the team with research experience and that the resources are available to them. Once this is established, you can further advocate for the team to not only act on best practices but also to begin adding to and improving best practices. Dr. Tim Porter-O'Grady and Dr. Kathy Malloch (2018) refer to this as recognizing evidence-based practice to be the "floor," or the starting point for clinical practice. Additional creativity and innovation, developed through Professional Governance Councils, allow the team to advance their clinical practice further, to the "ceiling." Skilled professional nurses working together in a learning environment can accomplish this type of advancement (American Organization of Nurse Executives, 2015; Porter-O'Grady & Malloch, 2018).

As you share your team's innovative solutions and practice changes across the organization, there will be a need for continued support and advocacy as solutions are adopted and changes are put in place. Measures of success must be established for all collaborating teams to bring about shared ownership and accountability.

Advocate in Action: Nurse managers often face an experience gap when transitioning seasoned staff and onboarding new nurses. Experienced nurses balance patient care and mentoring, while newer nurses work to meet expectations, affecting morale and leading to minor errors.

Collaborating with your director, you spotlight the issue with data and personal stories, shaping a strategy that includes:

- Reducing preceptors' patient loads to focus on mentorship.
- Floating experienced staff to stabilize high-demand shifts.
- Advocating for a Nurse Residency Support Coordinator.
- Hosting listening sessions to refine workflows and enhance learning.

Through empathy and consistent presence, you inspire confidence and foster growth, laying the groundwork for meaningful change.

The Awakener Meets Complexity

Porter-O'Grady and Malloch (2018), experts in complexity science and leadership, state that "aligning staff motivation with organizational goals is the only sustainable way of ensuring staff investment and ownership" (p. 147). Since we know that true motivation comes from within, you inspire motivation in individuals by aligning their inner desires with the work of the organization. This requires you to coach and mentor individuals rather than direct and delegate opportunities that will help individuals grow. It is through your coaching and mentoring, the team's work in Professional Governance Councils, and your advocacy that rich relationships are formed, and people self-organize and adapt to change. You, as an Awakener, encourage creativity and innovation by embracing the team's learning and any innovative surprises that emerge.

Outcomes Resulting from a Culture of Excellence

Journeys and roadmaps to excellence, such as the ANCC Magnet Recognition Program® and the American Nurses Credentialing Center (ANCC) Pathway to Excellence® Framework, describe the outcomes that attract and retain driven, compassionate nurses, and deliver market-leading results.

The Magnet Standards of Transformational Leadership; Structural Empowerment; Exemplary Professional Practice; and New Knowledge, Innovations, and Improvements are influenced by the leader embracing the dimension of the Awakener. See Appendix E for examples. As an Awakener focused on Magnet designation, you contribute to achieving goals such as fostering a culture of safety, implementing mentoring plans, enhancing RN satisfaction (including autonomy, interprofessional collaboration, and resource adequacy), reducing turnover, and improving patient outcomes. Additionally, you contribute to advancing evidence-based quality improvements, increasing certifications and BSN-prepared nurses, supporting effective role transitions, and developing individualized professional growth plans. These results stem from sustained attention to excellence rather than one-time efforts, reflecting your commitment to cultivating a thriving team and organization (refer to Appendix C).

The ANCC Pathway to Excellence Framework for Creating Positive Practice Environments (2020) also includes standards that rely on a Culture of Excellence.

> **Pathway Standard 6 (Professional Development)**: Recognizes the importance of solid onboarding, lifelong learning, ongoing education, and professional development to the delivery of safe and effective patient care. The foundation of developing competent and collaborative staff begins with a comprehensive orientation that includes individualization of learning needs. This ensures a smooth transition into practice. Guidance from mentors fosters the growth and development of emerging leaders essential for succession planning. Ensuring team members' professional growth and individual success leads to organizational success.
>
> **Pathway Standard 2 (Leadership)**: Ensures that nurse managers receive role-specific orientation and leaders equally strive to increase their core knowledge and role competency through leadership development activities, along with feedback from colleagues and nursing staff (refer to Appendix F).

From *Knowing* to *Doing*: Practical Ways to Influence a Culture of Excellence

Let's return to our framework of *Being-Knowing-Doing* to illustrate how to put the Awakener attributes into action. A culture of excellence emerges when values, mindset, and knowledge come together to drive meaningful action. This is how the Awakener moves from Being (values and mindset) to Knowing (knowledge) to Doing (meaningful action). While your core beliefs and principles lay the foundation, it is through intentional choices and behaviors that leaders truly shape their teams and environments. Actions that say "I believe in you" are grounded in the attributes of the Awakener. By motivating, coaching, mentoring, building a structure for growth, and advocating for the team's needs, the leader's actions lead to continuous learning and growth for the team and a commitment to continuous improvement in quality and patient safety. By aligning who you are with what you know and what you do, you become a catalyst for positive change, fostering a workplace where excellence thrives, and everyone feels empowered to contribute their best.

Create Individual Development Plans

As an Awakener, ensure that each nurse creates and owns their individual development plan, with you serving as a mentor, coach, and advocate for their growth. Goals within the plan should follow the S.M.A.R.T. format—specific, measurable, achievable, relevant, and time-based—and include professional growth, educational objectives, and activities to support self-care and mindfulness for enhanced resiliency and balance.

Collaborate with the nurse to identify required resources, measures of success, and target completion dates. While plans can align with organizational frameworks like ladder programs or pillars of excellence, they must be tailored to the unique needs of each individual. Regularly review and refine the plans during performance appraisals, celebrating milestones and achievements as they arise. Highlighting these accomplishments within the team fosters a culture of excellence and motivates continued development.

It's your turn to give it a try. Use the example provided below to guide your thoughts and ideas on writing a S.M.A.R.T. goal.

EXAMPLE

I will successfully pass the Certified Nurse Executive Advanced—Board Certification within three months by studying for the test content, completing the online practice test questions, and studying for 30 minutes, three times a week for the next three months.

Now, let's take it to the next level and consider personal and professional goals as well as goals to develop with our teams. Use the template (Table 3) to brainstorm ideas for yourself and with your team!

Celebrate Certified Nurses Day

This opportunity for recognition goes a long way in contributing to the motivation of team members. Certified Nurses Day occurs every March 19, the birthday of

S	M	A	R	T
SPECIFIC	**MEASURABLE**	**ATTAINABLE**	**REALISTIC**	**TIMELY**
What *specifically* do you want to do?	*How will you know* when you've achieved it?	Is it in your *power* to accomplish it?	Can you *realistically* achieve it?	When *exactly* do you want to accomplish it?

DRAFT YOUR GOAL:

TABLE 3 Individual Development Plan Template

Individual Long-Term Goal (3-5 years)					
S.M.A.R.T Goal	What resources are needed?	Who can help?	Review Date: Initial	Review Date: Follow-Up	Achieved Date
Individual Short-Term Goal (1-2 years)					
S.M.A.R.T Goal	What resources are needed?	Who can help?	Review Date: Initial	Review Date: Follow-Up	Achieved Date
Professional Goal					
Personal Goal					
Team Short-Term Goal (1-2 years)					
S.M.A.R.T Goal	What resources are needed?	Who can help?	Review Date: Initial	Review Date: Follow-Up	Achieved Date

Dr. Margretta "Gretta" Madden Styles, RN, EdD, FAAN, one of the greatest leaders in the field of nursing certification (ANCC, n.d.). To celebrate Certified Nurses Day, consider the following:

1. Post framed copies of the team members' certifications on the walls of the unit and celebrate milestones as the percentage of certified nurses on the unit increases.
2. Celebrate with a breakfast or lunch to recognize all certified nurses and provide information on certification to those not yet certified.

Develop a Peer Coaching Program

Peer coaching has been used in teacher education (Arslan Dönmez & Şahin, 2022; Golden, Hemmeter, Edmonds, & Ledford, 2021), medical education (Ackah et al., 2024; Mukherjee, LaCross, & Khalsa, 2024), and nursing education (Colón, 2024) for years but is gaining momentum in staff development and the clinical practice of bedside nurses and advance practice providers (Kramer, 2024). Peer coaching provides an opportunity for peers to practice newly learned skills and benefit from the nonhierarchical feedback of another learner. The intended benefits are quality improvement and risk reduction. According to Kramer (2024), peer coaching should be voluntary, and partners should be able to select each other. It should be used for the purpose of self-improvement and not as a part of an official performance review. In addition to the benefits of reflective practice and self-directed learning, peer coaching encourages true collegiality (Kramer, 2024).

1. Consider incorporating peer coaching in nurse residency programs.
2. Consider using peer coaching in programs designed for role transition.
3. What other opportunities are there in your organization for peer coaching?

Implement Visual Management Boards to Follow Quality Outcomes

Engage individual teams in identifying how they can contribute to a quality outcome. When teams determine their improvement processes, they take ownership of both the processes and outcomes. Lean management offers a helpful tool for managing changes, often referred to as "visual management" or a "performance board." These boards visually communicate improvement results to staff and leadership, fostering transparency and engagement.

Regular short huddles around the board provide insights into progress, support continuous learning, and create an informal space for shared governance where nurses can voice concerns and propose solutions. For example:

1. Use visual management boards to monitor new initiatives for improving nursing quality indicators, such as patient falls, pressure ulcers, central line-associated bloodstream infection, or catheter-associated urinary tract infection.
2. Strengthen team collaboration by encouraging shared leadership during daily huddles.

This approach not only drives improvements but also cultivates a collaborative environment where teams feel empowered to contribute meaningfully to quality outcomes.

Recognize a Just Culture Is a Safe Culture

Fostering a just culture within an organization requires shifting the focus from judging errors and outcomes to examining their origins. This approach emphasizes system design and behavioral choices, creating opportunities for learning and supporting caregivers through robust systems. By replacing the expectation of perfection with the goal of safe practices, a just culture balances accountability with psychological safety. It is neither punitive nor entirely blame-free but promotes professional responsibility while fostering a safer environment for both caregivers and patients, ultimately leading to better outcomes for families (Marx, 2019).

1. Celebrate team members who report near misses during unit or hospital safety huddles.
2. Refer near misses to the Professional Governance Council to develop innovative solutions for potential issues.

Discussion Questions for Groups

1. What are the metrics you currently follow to ensure a culture of excellence?
2. What structure do you have in place to encourage staff participation in innovative problem-solving?

3. As a leader, develop S.M.A.R.T. goals to improve your practice as the Awakener. Include goals and progress around the following: motivator, coach, mentor, architect, and advocate. Discuss your goals with your colleagues. How will you work together and harness the wisdom of the team? How can you help each other?
4. What do you need to move forward with creating and supporting professional development plans for your nurses?
5. How can you infuse the environment in your unit or department with the expectation of continuous growth and learning?
6. What resources do you have available to you to promote growth and learning among your staff? What else is needed?

Reflection Questions for Individuals

Think about your own professional growth and call to mind any leaders who acted as an Awakener by motivating, mentoring, and coaching you. How has this leader impacted your career and your life? Consider letting this leader know about their influence on your life. Recognizing people and thanking those who are important to you will contribute to your overall happiness and joy in life.

____

____

____

____

____

References

Ackah, R. L., Kenawy, D. M., Vaidya, P. S., Shalash, B. J., Haywood, K. T., Henry, R. C., . . . Chen, X. (2024). An assessment of barriers and facilitators of near-peer coaching on surgical clerkships: A mixed-methods study from residents' perspective. *Global Surgical Education, 3*, Article 62. https://link.springer.com/article/10.1007/s44186-024-00240-x

American Organization of Nurse Executives (2015, April 15). *Future of nursing: Empowering leaders igniting change* [Video]. YouTube. Retrieved from https://www.youtube.com/watch?v=ytAV0jcIVPc

Arslan Dönmez, S., & Şahin, A. (2022). Peer-coaching based professional development: A sample of a school of foreign languages. *Georgia Educational Researcher, 19*(1). https://digitalcommons.georgiasouthern.edu/gerjournal/vol19/iss1/2

Colón, E. F. (2024). Bridging the retention gap: An evaluation study of a peer coaching program for baccalaureate nursing students. Johns Hopkins University. https://jscholarship.library.jhu.edu/handle/1774.2/70102

Golden, A. K., Hemmeter, M. L., Edmonds, M., & Ledford, J. R. (2021). Reciprocal peer coaching and teaching teams' use of Pyramid Model practices. *Journal of Early Intervention, 43*(3), 255–274. doi: 10.1177/1053815121993225

Kramer, D. (2024). The importance of mentorship programs in nursing. In *A guide for developing a culture of caring through nursing peer mentorship programs*. Springer. doi: 10.1007/978-3-031-66139-6_1

Leclerc, L., Kennedy, K., & Campis, S. (2020). Human-centered leadership in healthcare: An idea that's time has come. *Nursing Administration Quarterly, 44*(2), 117–126.

Leclerc, L., Kennedy, K., & Campis, S. (2021). Human-centered leadership in healthcare: A contemporary nursing leadership theory generated via constructivist grounded theory. *Journal of Nursing Management, 29*(2), 294–306.

Marx, D. (2019). Patient safety and just culture. *Obstetrics and Gynecology Clinics of North America, 46*(2), 239–245. doi: 10.1016/j.ogc.2019.01.003

Mukherjee, B., LaCross, L., & Khalsa, G. (2024). A lifelong journey: A phenomenological exploration of faculty perceptions about coach training at an academic medical center. *BMC Medical Education, 24*, Article 1085. https://bmcmededuc.biomedcentral.com/articles/10.1186/s12909-024-06038-1

Porter-O'Grady, T., & Malloch, K. (2018). *Quantum leadership: Creating sustainable value in health care* (5th ed.). Jones & Bartlett.

Tye, J., & Dent, B. (2024). *Building a culture of ownership in healthcare: The invisible architecture of core values, attitude, and self-empowerment* (3rd ed.). Sigma Theta Tau International Honor Society of Nursing.

Recommended Reading

O'Donovan, R., Ward, M., De Brun, A., & McAuliffe, E. (2019). Safety culture in health care teams: A narrative review of the literature. *Journal of Nursing Management, 27*(5), 871–883. doi: 10.1111/jonm.12740

Schwellnus, H., & Carnahan, H. (2014). Peer-coaching with health care professionals: What is the current status of the literature and what are the key components necessary in peer-coaching? *Medical Teacher, 36*(1), 38–46.

Sherman, R. O. (2019). *The nurse leader coach: Become the boss no one wants to leave.* Rose O. Sherman.

Studer, Q. (2003). *Hardwiring excellence.* Fire Starter Publishing.

CHAPTER 8

The Connector

Creating a Culture of Trust

A leader is best when people barely know he exists,
when his work is done, his aim fulfilled, they will say:
we did it ourselves.

—Lao Tzu

The story below illustrates the human-centered leader's impact on the team within the complex system of healthcare. Specifically, you'll see how demonstrating the attributes of the Connector leads to a healthy work environment, a culture of trust, and engaged team members.

From Emojis to Impact—How Collaborative Problem-Solving Enhanced Patient Experience

Serving as the CNO of a large community hospital provided me with a unique opportunity to learn the importance of turning to experts for problem-solving. One such challenge involved addressing low scores on the patient experience survey, specifically regarding patients' understanding of their medications. It resulted in a solution that was initiated from *within* the organization rather than from the top. A manager in the pharmacy, Sabrina, was concerned about the fact that one question on the patient experience survey consistently received poor scores. It is related to the patient's understanding of the side effects of new medications. The exact question reads, "Before giving you any new medicine, how often did the hospital staff describe possible side effects in a way you could understand?" (U.S. Centers for Medicare and Medicaid Services, 2024). Sabrina thought there must be some way to improve this score, and she sincerely wanted the patients to be given information on their new medications. The problem seemed straightforward, especially since the nursing and pharmacy teams already had a strong working relationship. If it could be done, Sabrina thought the pharmacy and nursing teams could accomplish the improvement together.

Sabrina asked me for support and help in putting together a committee of interested nurse leaders and bedside caregivers. She was certain she could get her colleagues in the pharmacy involved. I was intrigued and excited about Sabrina's thoughts on collaborative problem-solving and went to work pulling together nurse leaders, nurse educators, and the patient experience team in preparation for the upcoming meeting. The nurse leaders were asked to bring any interested staff nurses along with them. The first meeting was designed to discuss the problem, consider barriers, and as time permitted, brainstorm possible solutions. In the first meeting, the team filled the boardroom, and I was witness to what Crowell (2016) describes as a "surprise" that emerged from the creativity of those intimately involved in self-organizing at the point of care.

One of the bedside nurses, a new graduate named Jermaine, attended the meeting. He had been a nurse for less than one year, yet he was tech-savvy and had previous experience working in graphic design and with teams. He spoke up, humbly offering a possible solution. Jermaine started by reviewing the problem as he saw it. He talked about issues such as health illiteracy, patients and staff members for whom English was their second or third language, and the ever-present concern in patient care of "information overload." There were also problems from the perspective of the nurses, such as time constraints and patients with numerous medications. Jermaine then pointed to a solution that he thought might address these barriers. He held up his laptop and began flipping through pages on his computer showing one screen after another of emojis representing different physical symptoms. One was green with nausea, another sported a big purple bruise, and still another had swirly, dizzy eyes. They all illustrated potential side effects of medications. His idea was to use the common language of emojis to communicate the side effects of medications to patients. He thought this would provide the patients with a clear understanding and be efficient for the nurses as well. Jermaine suggested that the nurse give the patient some type of small card to display the name of the medication and the emoji illustrations of the side effects. The patient could take the card home at discharge as a reminder of this important information.

The team was elated! This was indeed a creative solution. Others on the team joined in to add their creative ideas. Over the next couple of months, a graphic artist was hired, cards were designed for the most often prescribed medications, a system for storing and distributing the cards was developed, and the workflow for the staff was established. This solution, which came from a staff member, was much more sensitive to the barriers experienced at the point of care than any solutions that could have been developed by leaders at the top of the organization.

Unfortunately, the scores did not respond immediately to the change. There were problems with the new workflow resulting in inconsistencies among caregivers. In addition, some medications didn't have an associated side-effects card because those meds weren't in the top tier of "most commonly prescribed medications." Despite the challenges, each discipline worked to fine-tune their part of the process and make this seemingly simple solution a part of the normal, but complex, workflow.

After a few months, solid and consistent improvement in the patient experience scores followed, and the team was invited to present the project at the annual national meeting for Press Ganey, the industry's recognized leader in patient experience. This was a professional "high" for the team as they received many accolades for the success of their collaborative and innovative solution.

This story exemplifies the complexity of the healthcare organization, due to their interconnectedness and unpredictability. The team self-organized. The pharmacy, the nursing staff, and the patient experience team were all intricately connected, and this solution emerged from their collective wisdom. All I had to do was provide the environment for the solution to emerge, to be explored, and to be sustained. In a situation such as this, when the solution comes from within, there is no need for micromanaging, "holding the team accountable," or overreacting to inconsistencies in the data. The team makes it happen. As a result, they are accountable for the outcomes, and they are to be recognized for their creative solution.

Start with Self: *Be* the Connector

Leadership that fosters unity, trust, and innovation begins with self-awareness. To be the kind of leader who engages others, embraces diverse perspectives, and empowers creative problem-solving, your values and mindset must serve as the foundation. Start by examining your core values—trustworthiness, humility, curiosity, and respect—all of which shape the way you lead and build connections. A leader who cultivates trust doesn't hesitate to seek solutions from the team, amplify individual strengths, or create space for collaboration. Do your team members feel supported? Do they know you are in their corner, championing their ideas? Are they encouraged to think creatively and take ownership of solutions? When your values are consistently reflected in your behaviors, they become contagious—sparking engagement, deepening trust, and strengthening the fabric of the team.

Developing the Mindset of the Connector: I Don't Have to Have All the Answers

Leadership isn't about having all the answers—it's about creating the conditions where others can thrive. The mindset of the Connector begins with a pivotal shift: recognizing that your role as a leader isn't to solve every problem but to empower those around you to do so. This requires humility and trust—qualities that enable you to champion your team's expertise and foster an environment where innovation flourishes. Many leaders rise by being problem-solvers, yet true leadership emerges when they shift from knowing to enabling—celebrating their team's success, amplifying contributions, and strengthening the collective vision.

As you deepen your understanding of the Connector, you move from Being—your core values and beliefs—to Knowing, where knowledge and insight shape how you empower others. Unlike traditional leadership models that emphasize control and individual achievement, relational leadership is rooted in trust and shared success. Think back to a moment when a leader placed their trust in you—how did it shape your confidence and engagement? When leaders build trust and inspire collaboration, they don't just guide teams; they cultivate movements fueled by purpose, curiosity, and the boundless potential of empowered minds (Figure 5).

The Language of the Connector—"I trust you"

The language of the Connector—"I trust you"—is more than just words; it's a powerful catalyst for building genuine connections and fostering team empowerment. When backed by meaningful actions—inviting collaboration, encouraging innovation, supporting team ownership, and recognizing the unique strengths of each person—this phrase becomes truly transformative. Leaders who consistently show trust in their

FIGURE 5
The Connector.

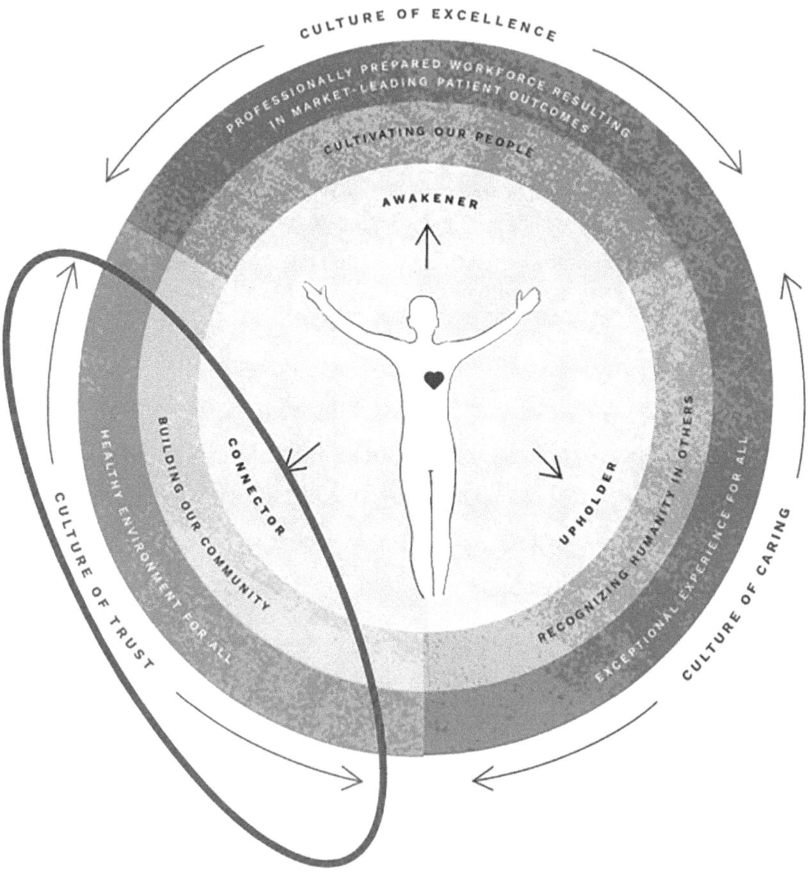

Note: Adapted from Leclerc, Kennedy, and Campis (2021).

teams create an environment where people feel engaged, valued, and inspired to take ownership of their work. In the sections ahead, we'll explore these actions in depth and uncover the key attributes that define the Connector.

Bring Unity to the Team Through *Knowing*

The attributes of the Connector include supporter, collaborator, edgewalker, engineer, and authentic communicator (see Table 4). By embracing these attributes, you, as the leader, demonstrate your belief in the team and their ability to unite around the mission, vision, and values of the organization. A quote from McChrystal, Collins, Silverman, and Fussell (2015) sums up the leader's role as a Connector:

TABLE 4 Defined Attributes Embodied by the Human-Centered Leader as a Connector

Connector	Builds our community
Collaborator	Unifies others around shared mission and vision.
Supporter	Supports, recognizes, and appreciates individual contributions.
Edgewalker	Embraces change by supporting experimentation of ideas to generate innovative solutions.
Engineer	Ensures people are positioned within teams to leverage their individual strengths while enhancing overall team performance.
Authentic Communicator	Builds mutual trust through authentic presence, active listening, and speaking with integrity.

Note: Adapted from Leclerc, Kennedy, and Campis (2021).

> "The temptation to lead as a chess master, controlling each move of the organization, must give way to an approach as a gardener, enabling rather than directing. A gardening approach to leadership is anything but passive. The leader acts as an 'Eyes-On, Hands-Off' enabler who creates and maintains an ecosystem in which the organization operates." (Collins, Silverman, & Fussell, 2015, p. 232).

As you learn more about the attributes of the Connector in the sections below, pay attention to how real-world nurses and healthcare leaders bring them to life in practice. We present selected examples and quotations from our original research, which have been substantiated through continuous investigation over the past several years.

Collaborator

When you think about collaboration, do you primarily envision working with other leaders across the organization? While that's undeniably important, don't overlook the opportunity to collaborate with your own team. Human-centered leaders position themselves within the team rather than above it. From this vantage point—at the heart of the work—you can listen deeply, understand their needs, remove obstacles, and tap into their creativity and capabilities to solve problems. As a Connector, your role is to unite the team around the mission, vision, and values of the organization. Simply put, the Connector brings unity to the community! And the most effective way to bring people together is through collaboration. The more diverse your team, the greater the potential impact—each person's unique strengths can become a driving force for innovation and success.

In our research, nurses described the leader they would "follow to the ends of the earth" as someone who collaborates by *identifying the goal and providing meaningful support* along the way. These leaders show genuine interest in their team members' work and abilities. The nurses referred to them as *opinion seekers*—leaders who practice appreciative inquiry and eagerly gather insight from different perspectives. More than anything, these nurses valued leaders who *truly listened, acknowledged their contributions, and provided choices when possible.* They felt honored and supported, knowing their decisions were respected. One nurse even noted that their *leader respects the analytical nature of team members*, highlighting the importance of understanding and appreciating diverse approaches to problem-solving.

Collaborator in Action: Josie, a nurse leader in critical care, was faced with a problem with patient flow. The busy ED in a large public hospital was not able to move patients to the ICU promptly. Even after the bed was assigned, giving report and transporting the critical patient were taking too long. Josie learned of a similar hospital that made progress on this issue by having the ICU nurse go to the ED for bedside handoff and then transport the patient to their ICU bed. As you might guess, the ICU staff was not in favor of this idea. Josie met with both teams together every week, listened to their different perspectives, asked for their ideas, and supported their progress. Josie kept the focus on the common goal of improving the care from the patient's perspective. After a couple of months, the teams began to collaborate with each other. They developed a handoff tool and established a process to address problems in real time. Josie modeled collaboration for the team, and in time, they began to collaborate. It took time to build trust, respect, and establish relationships. It required each team to understand the perspective of the other side. Josie was successful in her collaborative efforts, but more importantly, the patients were better served because of the unity between the teams and individuals.

Supporter

What does it truly mean to support your team and its members? If you've ever had a leader who genuinely supported you, you've likely felt empowered, secure, respected, and trusted. These feelings of validation create the freedom to perform at your best. When leaders offer authentic support, fear fades, and learning from mistakes becomes an opportunity rather than a setback. In this space, people feel free to stretch, create, and innovate. As you support your team, your trust in their expertise and abilities unlocks their sense of empowerment. In turn, they may surprise you with their creativity, problem-solving skills, and ability to foster a healthy, collaborative environment.

In our research, nurses described leaders with Connector traits as those who openly *demonstrate their confidence in the team and trust that the work will be done.* These leaders are consistently kind to individuals and deeply understand that "each person is fighting their own battles." By embodying this kind of trust, compassion, and belief in their team, leaders create an environment where people feel truly valued and motivated to contribute their best work.

Supporter in Action: The manager of an ICU, José, was concerned about the increase in CLABSIs among their critical patients. He met with the nurses on the unit and clearly shared with them his concerns about the trend in these data. He humbly stated that he did not have the answers, but he was confident in the team's ability to determine any gaps in care and develop a solution to this patient safety concern. He trusted their expertise and knowledge and was there to support their efforts. The team worked together in their Professional Governance Council, researched best practices, and developed innovative solutions. They sought out a superior central line dressing for their patient population. They also established a "buddy system" to use during sterile central line dressing changes to ensure compliance with the dressing change checklist. José's support allowed the team the freedom to explore viable solutions, which led to improved patient outcomes by decreasing the number of CLABSIs. In addition, José's support reinforced their confidence in their abilities to innovate and improve care.

Edgewalker

An *edgewalker*, as defined by Neal (2021), is someone who navigates the space between two worlds with distinct perspectives on organizational leadership. One world represents traditional leadership, while the other embraces a more contemporary, complexity-driven approach—like Human-Centered Leadership. Balancing both is essential to maintaining key processes while remaining open to unpredictability and change. Without uncertainty, innovation and progress wouldn't be possible.

The nurses in our research described edgewalkers as leaders who *bring their team along* on the journey. These leaders excel at gaining staff buy-in and have a natural ability to see and *communicate the bigger picture.* Rather than dictating the process, they immerse themselves in it, *fostering collaboration and openness.* They embrace the unexpected contributions of creative individuals and teams, welcoming fresh ideas and unconventional solutions. Most importantly, they *value and appreciate people who think differently.*

The Edgewalker in Action: Cindy, a nurse leader challenged with the goal of preparing bedside staff for the upcoming Joint Commission triannual visit, brought together a team of nurse educators and clinical nurse specialists to work together on this project. Cindy explained to the team that there was concern among the executive team that bedside nurses were not aware of new regulatory requirements. In the past, this would have required massive audits to determine nurses' gaps in knowledge, followed by education sessions, and then repeated audits. The team thought there must be a better way. Cindy was completely open and welcomed new, creative ideas. Through brainstorming and synergy, the team decided to develop a Joint Commission information fair. They identified the areas that nurses needed to learn about and developed games to teach the new information. They set up a "fair" and developed a schedule that allowed every nurse to attend. The nurses played Jeopardy, Go Fish, and Password. They easily learned the new regulations, in a new way, and the Joint Commission survey was highly successful! Cindy was an edgewalker who was willing to risk a new, creative approach to solving a problem that carried a high risk.

Engineer

As an engineer, the Connector takes a big-picture approach, thoughtfully integrating team members into the process in a way that recognizes and values their strengths. Once you, as the leader, establish a shared understanding of each team member's role, your responsibility—according to our research participants—is to *allow, support, and expect autonomy.* When given the space to own their work, team members embrace their empowerment and confidently contribute toward the goal. With accountability built into the process, there's no need for micromanaging—just trust in the team's ability to deliver.

Engineer in Action: Think back to the story about Jermaine and the collaborative team who developed the cards with medication side effects illustrated through the common language of emojis. Each member of the team worked in the area of their strength. Pharmacists worked on the list of the most commonly prescribed medications and side effects, nurse educators worked on establishing and teaching the workflow, and the patient experience team members worked with the graphic artist to bring the design to life. As this team evolved and the excitement grew, others wanted to be involved in the work. Executive assistants jumped in to work on the logistics of purchasing the storage boxes and ordering supplies. Each team member generously gave their time and expertise and worked autonomously in their area of strength, and the entire team succeeded as a result.

Authentic Communicator

Authentic communication is easy to recognize—and ironically, the best way to demonstrate it is through engaged listening. When you truly listen, you build meaningful connections. The nurses in our research described authentic communication as *forthright, transparent, and free from politics*—a genuine two-way conversation where diverse perspectives are welcomed.

By honing your conflict resolution skills, you show your commitment to open dialogue and mutual respect. This fosters a *safe environment* where team members feel empowered to express themselves. Authenticity also means *being honest, demonstrating integrity, earning trust, and respecting every person on the team.* Follow through on your commitments and honor confidentiality—because integrity isn't just about words; it's about actions. And one simple rule to live by? *Don't gossip.*

Authentic Communicator in Action: Every year, Lisa, the nurse manager of an ICU, knew her team would take the employee engagement survey, and she would be required to develop an action plan around their responses. Even though Lisa had a good relationship with her team, she always worried a bit about what their comments would reveal. Did they think she was doing a good job? Were there problems on the unit she wasn't aware of? The time came and the survey results were in. Thankfully, most of the comments about the work environment were positive, but there was a consistent negative comment about Lisa. Team members thought that she played favorites. Lisa was quite upset because she had no idea that she was giving this impression. She called a staff meeting to develop an action plan. As the meeting progressed, the discussion turned to Lisa and the issue of favoritism. Lisa listened carefully, and with empathy, to the staff. She was able to see the situation through their eyes, and she genuinely apologized for her lack of external self-awareness. She spoke from the heart about her intentions and her desire to engage completely with each of them in an equitable manner. She committed that she would do her best to change this perception and asked the team in return to commit to letting her know if they noticed a problem. Lisa's authentic communication proved to be an opportunity for further trust and connection between her and the team.

The Connector Meets Complexity

The attributes of the Connector clearly link the human-centered leader to the foundations of complexity science and complex adaptive systems. Remember Jermaine and his team who developed the emoji cards to influence patient outcomes and satisfaction? Jermaine's story illustrates that connected workgroups, united in their pursuit of the organization's mission and vision, can create innovative solutions. How does that happen? Is it predictable? Carmichael and Hadžikadić (2019) outline the parameters of complex adaptive systems, which are recognizable in our story: information flows freely; there is rich connectivity; there are diverse mental models; there is diversified leadership; and there are simple rules. The team was given free rein to create a solution to the problem around patients' understanding of the side effects of their new medications. The members shared their different perspectives and connected processes. The rules were simple—no constraints were put in place. The leadership was diversified as team members gravitated toward their individual areas of strength. The stage was set for self-organization and innovation. Creative ideas, like the one Jermaine shared, emerge from within a complex system and can have a huge impact on the organization. The proposed solution by a new nurse graduate produced what is known in complexity science as the "butterfly effect." His small contributions resulted in big outcomes for the organization.

Outcomes Resulting from a Culture of Trust

According to the Great Place to Work (n.d.) model, the values of credibility, respect, and fairness create **trust**. When you act as a Connector, you demonstrate these values through authentic communication, support, collaboration, plugging people into the appropriate structures for collaborative problem-solving (engineer), and extending trust to the team by encouraging innovation around change and unpredictability (edgewalker). The American Association of Critical Care Nurses (AACN, 2021) describes this type of trusting culture as a "healthy work environment." There is an extensive body of nursing research on the criteria for developing healthy work environments and the associated positive outcomes for nurses and patients. To put it simply, nurses who work in trusting environments are more fulfilled in their work, and their patients receive safe, high-quality care. As you practice the attributes of the Connector, your leadership skills will contribute to a culture of trust and your outcomes will align closely with those required by the ANCC Magnet Recognition Program standards (2023) and the ANCC Pathway to Excellence standards (2020).

The Magnet Standards of Transformational Leadership, Structural Empowerment, Exemplary Professional Practice, and New Knowledge, Innovations and Improvements are influenced by the leader embracing the dimension of the Connector. See Appendix E for examples. As a Connector focused on achieving Magnet designation, you contribute to achieving outcomes such as advancing culturally sensitive and population health initiatives, fostering nurse and interprofessional collaboration to achieve strategic goals, enhancing RN satisfaction and teamwork, decreasing turnover rates, driving research, and implementing patient-centered improvements informed by feedback. Achieving these outcomes reflects the work of a human-centered leader who embodies the attributes of the Connector (refer to Appendix C).

The ANCC Pathway to Excellence Framework for Creating Positive Practice Environments (2020) also includes standards that rely on a Culture of Trust. These standards include:

Pathway Standard 1 (Shared Decision-Making): Encourage and embrace input from direct care nurses and other disciplines in making decisions that impact care delivery. Interprofessional collaboration is integral to engaging staff, building teamwork, and strengthening the shared governance culture.

Pathway Standard 4 (Quality): Ensure that staff are aligned with the organization's mission, vision, values, and goals. Direct care nurses are involved in the review and implementation of evidence-based practice (refer to Appendix F).

From *Knowing* to *Doing*: Practical Ways to Influence a Culture of Trust

Let's revisit our framework of *Being-Knowing-Doing* to explore how the Connector brings the attributes to life. A culture of trust takes shape when values, mindset, and knowledge align to inspire purposeful action. This is how the Connector transitions from Being (values and mindset) to Knowing (knowledge) to Doing (purposeful action). Core beliefs and principles lay the groundwork, but it is through deliberate choices and behaviors that leaders truly shape their teams and environment. For the Connector, actions that convey "I trust you" are foundational. By fostering collaboration, supporting ownership, exploring innovative ideas, highlighting individual strengths, and demonstrating authenticity through "walking the talk," leaders empower their teams to take charge of both processes and outcomes.

Trust becomes the bedrock for achieving meaningful results. When leaders align their values, expertise, and actions, they transform into catalysts for positive change. This alignment fosters a workplace where trust is not just a concept but a lived experience—one where team members feel safe, valued, and fully invested in their work.

Everyday Practices of a Connector: Empowering Teams Through Trust

Ensure Team's Voice in Hiring: Leaders collaborate with stakeholders, i.e., human resources, to ensure policy and practice are aligned for direct care nurses to provide input in the hiring process for new staff. (Collaborator)

Elevate Evidence-Based Practice: Leaders support and recognize individual and collective contributions to safe, quality patient care grounded in evidence-based practice. This could occur through the leader providing resources to implement a project such as changes in patient OR prep for vaginal procedures using Association of periOperative Nurses (AORN) guidelines. (Supporter)

Prioritize Safety in the Work Environment: Leaders create a culture of trust where psychological and physical safety are prioritized to mitigate workplace violence; provide consistent and persistent messaging to team members that their physical and psychological well-being will be protected. (Authentic Communicator)

Ask for Staffing Input: Leaders embrace input from direct care nurses about daily staffing decisions by providing a safe psychological space in which innovation can emerge, i.e., huddles (unit and entity level), and validated acuity tools. (Edgewalker)

Build on Team Members' Strengths: Leaders look for strengths and opportunities to leverage strengths in practice. Encourage self-reflection. Reward and recognize individuals for their strengths and positive results. (Engineer)

Embrace AACN's (2021) Standards for a Healthy Work Environment

AACN (2021) provides standards required for a healthy work environment: authentic communication, true collaboration, effective decision-making, appropriate staffing, meaningful recognition, and authentic leadership (refer to Appendix H).

1. Ask your team to take the AACN Healthy Work Environment assessment to determine strengths and areas for improvement. The assessment is available on the AACN website (https://www.aacn.org/nursing-excellence/healthy-work-environments).
2. Ask team members to work through Professional Governance on specific strategies to improve the work environment.
3. Embrace VitalSmarts, *Silence Kills*, an industry study, and support the team in practicing crucial conversations (Maxfield, Grenny, McMillan, Patterson, & Switzler, 2005).
4. Recognize the strengths individual team members possess and plug these members into the Professional Governance and other committee opportunities to leverage their strengths.
5. Work with your team to determine how to best reward and recognize those who are excelling and contributing to the mission, vision, and values of the unit and organization.
6. Foster a culture of respect and inclusion while addressing and preventing bullying behaviors.
7. Make respect for each other a palpable value in the workplace.
8. Engage team members in developing creative staffing models to meet the needs of patients and leverage staff working collaboratively and at "top of license."
9. Trust your team and the decisions made through Professional Governance.
10. What other ways can you support the development of a healthy work environment?

____

____

____

____

____

Discussion Questions for Groups

1. Which staff members are involved in your Professional Governance Councils? Are your teams diverse and inclusive? Are people plugged into the areas where their strengths shine?
2. Is your team involved in any research around improving clinical practice? How can you support this process?
3. How has your team collaborated across the system? Is there a structure in place to ensure this communication and collaboration occurs?
4. Does your team see you as an edgewalker? How do you demonstrate to the team that you are open to change and innovation? How do you embrace unpredictability?

Reflection for Individuals

Consider taking the AACN Healthy Work Environment assessment available on the AACN website (AACN, 2021). As you review the results, reflect on your own experiences within your work environment. What aspects contribute positively to your well-being and effectiveness? Where do you notice challenges that may need attention? What intentional actions can you take to foster a healthier, more supportive workplace?

____

____

____

____

____

References

American Association of Critical Care Nurses. (2021). *AACN standards for establishing and sustaining healthy work environments: Journey to excellence* (2nd ed.). Retrieved from https://www.aacn.org/nursing-excellence/healthy-work-environments

Carmichael, T., & Hadžikadić, M. (2019). The fundamentals of complex adaptive systems. In T. Carmichael, A. Collins, & M. Hadžikadić (Eds.), *Complex adaptive systems: Understanding complex systems.* Springer. doi: 10.1007/978-3-030-20309-2_1

Centers for Medicare and Medicaid Service. (2024). Updated HCAHPS survey. Retrieved from https://hcahpsonline.org/en/updated-hcahps-survey/

Crowell, D. M. (2016). *Complexity leadership* (2nd ed.). FA Davis Co.

Great Place to Work. (n.d.). *The definition of a great workplace*. Retrieved from www.greatplacetowork.com/trustmodel#:~:text=The%20Employee%20View%3A%20The%20Great%20Place%20to%20Work%C2%AE,the%20foundation%20of%20our%20Trust%20Index%C2%A9%20Employee%20Survey

Leclerc, L., Kennedy, K., & Campis, S. (2021). Human-centered leadership in healthcare: A contemporary nursing leadership theory generated via constructivist grounded theory. *Journal of Nursing Management, 29*(2), 294–306.

Maxfield, D., Grenny, J., McMillan, R., Patterson, K., & Switzler, A. (2005). *Silence kills: The seven crucial conversations for healthcare*. VitalSmarts Industry Watch. Retrieved from https://www.aacn.org/nursing-excellence/healthy-work-environments/~/media/aacn-website/nursing-excellence/healthy-work-environment/silencekills.pdf?la=en

McChrystal, S., Collins, T., Silverman, D., & Fussell, C. (2015). *Team of teams: New rules of engagement for a complex world.* Penguin.

Neal, J. (2021). *Creating edgewalker organizations.* Edgewalkers. Retrieved from https://edgewalkers.org/resources/articles-by-judi-neal/351-2

Recommended Reading

Patterson, K., Grenny, J., McMillan, J., & Switzler, A. (2004). *Crucial confrontations: Tools for resolving broken promises, violated expectations, and bad behavior*. McGraw Hill.

Patterson, K., Grenny, J., McMillan, R., & Switzler, A. (2008). *Influencer: The power to change anything.* McGraw Hill.

Patterson, K., Grenny, J., McMillan, R., & Switzler, A. (2012). *Crucial conversations: Tools for talking when stakes are high* (2nd ed.). McGraw Hill.

Thompson, R. (2013). *"Do no harm" applies to nurses too*! Incredible Messages Press.

Thompson, R. (2019). *Enough! Eradicate bullying and incivility in healthcare*. Incredible Messages Press.

CHAPTER 9

The Upholder

Cultivating a Culture of Caring

Take care of your people, and they will take care of the mission.

—James Mattis, Retired four-star general
of the United States Marine Corps
and a former U.S. Secretary of Defense

Some leaders have a special ability to genuinely care for their team—not in a way that feels overbearing or controlling, but more like a supportive colleague or trusted friend. These leaders prioritize both their own well-being and that of others, fostering an environment where people feel valued and empowered. Their focus is not just on leadership—it's on inspiring individuals to co-create a culture of caring.

From Resistance to Resilience: An Upholder's Leadership Legacy

When Evalyn, a seasoned nurse leader, joined the leadership team at her new organization, she encountered an uphill battle. The staff were not at all receptive to her. They feared that she wouldn't "advocate" for them, that she was "on the side of management," and that she had never "walked in their shoes." They wondered how she could understand their perspective. Evalyn had not risen from the ranks of the organization. She was from the "outside" and this, in and of itself, created a sense of uncertainty among the team. They didn't know what changes she might put in place and, more importantly, how those changes might impact them. Even as Evalyn was keenly aware of the team's attitude toward her, she stayed focused on her intention to strengthen the team by first embracing them and creating a culture where the team members authentically cared for each other and for their patients. Looking back, I realize that it was her emotional intelligence that allowed her to stay calm rather than become defensive, remain self-assured and self-confident in her leadership methods, and continually reach out to establish and manage relationships. One crucial key to her success was that she *always* gave the team credit for accomplishments, which reinforced her support and confidence in them and, in time, helped them trust her.

Evalyn went about leading this team in a mindful, calm, and poised manner. She wore scrubs and worked alongside the staff whenever possible. She got to know the staff members as individuals. After a while, the staff realized that her engagement with them involved her full attention on their humanness, their strengths, and their good intentions. Evalyn is not one to blame or shame. Instead, she pulled the team together around their mission—patient safety and excellent patient care.

At the same time, Evalyn was no pushover. She held a high bar for engagement and service excellence and had to make the tough decision to terminate a few staff members who were not willing to fully engage in the work. Some staff members self-selected out once they realized that the expectations had changed and, for whatever reason, they were not willing or able to make a change themselves. Evalyn held a high bar for engagement, service, and civility, and by doing so, she further endorsed the standards of the unit and created a culture of caring. She lived by the rule that leaders must hold high moral standards and follow ethical guidelines when addressing any disrespectful or disruptive behavior. At the same time, Evalyn ensured that staff were validated and rewarded for exemplary commitment to the values of the organization (Fulford & Coleman, 2021; Hernandez & Summers, 2024). By consistently modeling the organization's values and recognizing others for demonstrating those same values, Evalyn's leadership led to a culture of caring.

How did she do it? Evalyn is one of those people who are naturally curious about other people. She wants to know what motivates them, how they relate to the world, and what their values are. She demonstrated her values by being present, in mind and body, which allowed her to establish open, trusting relationships. She consistently rounded on all the staff and the patients, listening to their concerns, and responding with empathy and compassion. The staff recognized that it wasn't just the patients who mattered, nor was it just the metrics—it was them, the team. She was authentic in her actions. She could be counted on to mean and do what she said she would and to extend authentic caring to each staff member, patient, and family. Her actions demonstrated what Goleman, Boyatzis, and McKee (2013) described as "gifted leadership"—where the heart and the head meet.

As a result of Evalyn's leadership, the team became more engaged with each other, with their colleagues from other disciplines, and with their patients. Their engagement score moved up a tier on an organization-wide survey, and their patient experience scores topped out at the 99th percentile. The turnover rate decreased, and the unit was known to be a place where nurses wanted to work. Whenever an administrator, physician, nurse, or VIP was admitted to the hospital, they were admitted to this unit. Why? Because the unit's reputation was that patients received excellent care and the nursing staff was outstanding. These outcomes came about from a culture change—from the leadership behaviors attributed to the qualities of the Upholder, not from a newly established organization-wide initiative.

Start with Self: *Be* the Upholder

To foster an environment where people feel genuinely cared for, a leader's core values and mindset become the driving force. The guiding values grounding the dimension of the Upholder are wellness, inclusivity, dignity, humility, and empathy. These values allow leaders to cultivate fairness and compassion, ensuring every individual feels seen, valued, and understood. As discussed earlier, your values and mindset shape your intentions and become evident in your actions. If your goal is to inspire care and compassion among the team which overflows to the patients in their care, start with reflecting on your values as a leader. It starts with you!

Cultivating the Mindset of an Upholder: Inclusion

Creating inclusivity and belonging begins with a leader's commitment to self-reflection and growth. By examining personal biases and assumptions, leaders open the door to greater understanding and empathy. Listening actively to team members' experiences and perspectives fosters deeper connections and helps build trust. Leaders who embrace continuous learning—about cultural, social, and individual differences—create an environment that celebrates diversity and encourages open, meaningful dialogue. Moreover, modeling inclusivity through genuine actions and transparent behavior sets a powerful example for others to follow. When leaders seek input from all team members, they create a space where every voice matters. Finally, recognizing and honoring the unique contributions of individuals strengthens mutual respect and a shared sense of belonging, creating a culture where everyone feels valued and supported.

As you deepen your understanding of the Upholder and transition from *being* to *knowing*, remember that your ultimate goal is to bring the values of wellness, inclusivity, dignity, humility, and empathy into your actions. Gaining a better understanding of the attributes of the Upholder will help you do just that (Figure 6).

FIGURE 6
The Upholder.

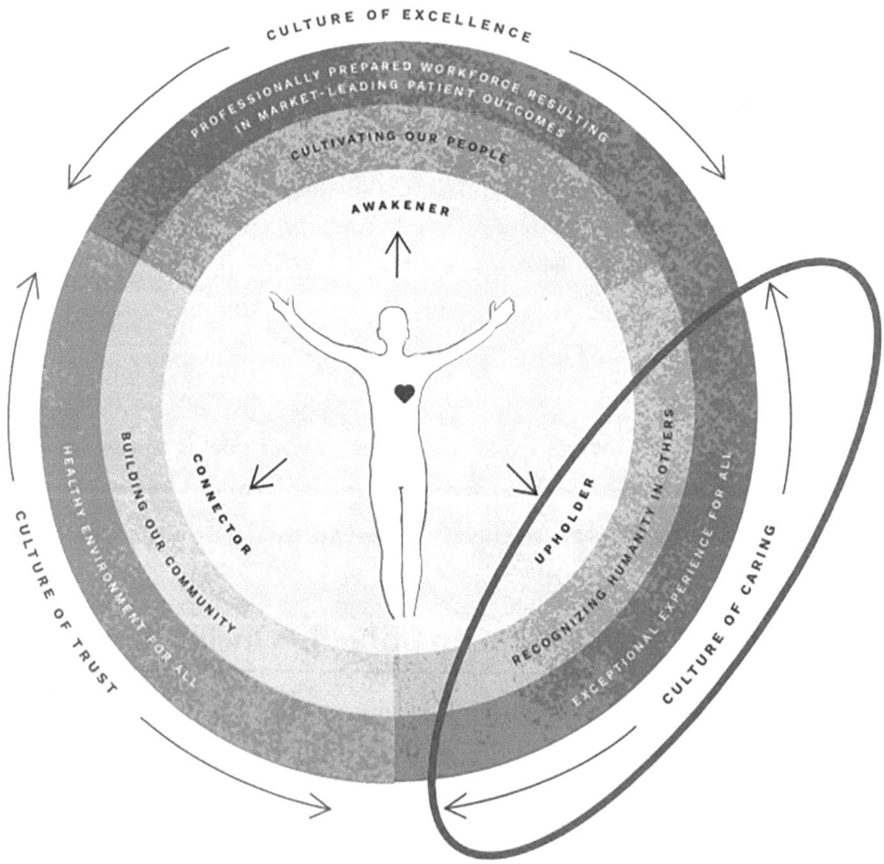

Note: Adapted from Leclerc et al. (2021).

The Language of the Upholder—"I see you."

The Upholder embodies inclusivity and belonging through a simple yet powerful phrase: *"I see you."* But what does it truly mean in practice?

It starts with active listening—being fully present in conversations, maintaining focus, and responding thoughtfully to show genuine engagement. Leaders can further strengthen connections by recognizing individual contributions through personalized praise or public acknowledgment, ensuring every team member feels valued.

Empathy plays a crucial role, too. Acknowledging emotions and offering support during challenges fosters trust and connection. Beyond professional interactions, remembering personal details and holding regular one-on-one check-ins demonstrate deep care and attentiveness. Together, these thoughtful actions reinforce a culture of caring through nurturing belonging and mutual respect. The outcome results in an environment where everyone feels truly seen and appreciated.

Uphold Others Through *Knowing*

The attributes of the Upholder are personally well and healthy, mindful, others-oriented, emotionally aware, and socially and organizationally aware (Table 5). As you learn more about the attributes of the Upholder in the sections below, pay attention to how real-world nurses and healthcare leaders bring them to life in practice. We've included a few examples and quotes from our original research that have been confirmed through ongoing exploration in recent years.

TABLE 5 Defined Attributes Embodied by the Human-Centered Leader as an Upholder

Upholder	**Recognizes humanity in others**
Mindful	Focuses attention, awareness, and energy on the present.
Others-Oriented	Supports with respect, kindness, empathy, and empowerment.
Emotionally Aware	Recognizes how emotions influence behavior, communication, and relationships.
Socially and Organizationally Aware	Recognizes context, unwritten rules, and unspoken words to guide interactions.
Personally Well and Healthy	Prioritizes harmony between work and personal life demands to empower others to do the same.

Note: Adapted from Leclerc, Kennedy, and Campis (2021).

Mindful

Nurses in our research emphasized the profound impact of mindfulness, recognizing it through *openness and presence*—the ability to truly *listen* and respond with *empathy* and *understanding*. They spoke about leaders who *treated them like a person* and *related to their experiences*, fostering trust and connection.

Chang, Donald, Whitney, Miao, and Sahdra (2023) suggest that mindfulness helps individuals release bias, preconceptions, judgments, and expectations, creating space for authentic engagement. The leader as an Upholder embraces this practice, actively valuing diversity and inclusivity within the team. By approaching interactions with curiosity rather than assumptions, they cultivate an environment where every team member feels respected, seen, and heard (Leclerc et al., 2021).

Emotionally Aware

In addition, the nurses participating in our research talked about the emotional intelligence required of leaders. Emotional intelligence helps leaders *build relationships*, *be respectful*, and *appreciate humanity in others*. It is emotional intelligence that allows the leader to recognize and understand emotions in themselves and others and to use this awareness to manage behaviors and relationships (Bradberry & Greaves, 2009).

Others-Oriented

The nurses in our research study talked about leaders who were *others-oriented*. They described an outward focus that could be described as *empathy*, *advocacy*, *supportiveness*, and *compassion*. One nurse said that the *leader reflected the staff, rather than the staff reflecting the leader*. This likely means that each staff member felt highly valued and understood by the leader because they experienced an others-oriented approach to leadership.

When you think about the term "others-oriented," does it bring to mind the value of compassion? Do you think about a leader's positive intentions and real concern for the well-being of others? While this is a correct description of compassion, understand that compassion alone is not enough. For effective leadership, compassion must be combined with wisdom. *Wise compassion* is the ability to do hard things in a human way. It means you can make hard decisions, give tough feedback, and when necessary, even lay off members of your team. Wise compassion means you balance concern for others with the need to move the organization forward in an effective manner (Hougaard, Carter, & Hobson, 2020). If you've ever had to lay someone off and they responded positively with a "thank you," and maybe even a hug, you've probably got the right balance. If not, read on. . . .

If you need more compassion to get the right balance, remember to embrace the other attributes of the Upholder—practice mindfulness and become intentionally aware of others' emotions. Start with yourself and practice self-compassion. Check your intentions before you have a direct and difficult conversation. Set your intention to provide a benefit to others. Lastly, practice compassion daily so it will become a habit for you (Hougaard et al., 2020).

On the other hand, if you tend to weigh in heavier on the side of compassion, practice candid transparency. Remember your intention is to benefit others. Concealing criticism is misleading. Brené Brown (2018) is known for saying, "Being clear is kind.

The Mindful, Emotionally Aware, and Others-Oriented Leader in Action

Jean Watson (2009), theorist and expert in the "Art of Caring," suggests the following ways to demonstrate **"Caring in Action,"** which correlate with these attributes of the Upholder:

- Creating intentional and meaningful rituals. For example, hand washing is for infection control but also may be a meaningful ritual of self-care and mindfulness.
- Creating healing spaces for nurses: sanctuaries for their time out. May include meditation or relaxation rooms for quiet time.
- Intentionally pausing and breathing. For example, preparing myself to be present before entering patients' rooms.
- Selecting caring-healing modalities for self and patients. For example, massage, therapeutic touch, reflexology, aromatherapy, sound, music, arts, and a variety of energetic modalities.
- Dimming the unit lights and having designated "quiet time" for patients, families, and staff, to soften, slow down, and calm the environment.
- Engaging in caring rounds at patients' bedsides. For example, focus on non-physical aspects of care such as spiritual and emotional needs.
- Engaging in centering exercises and mindfulness practices as a group. For example, add a mindful moment to huddles (Watson, 2009).

Being unclear is unkind." Try to practice having a direct and assertive interaction every day so you can make *wise compassion* a habit (Hougaard et al., 2020).

Socially and Organizationally Aware

The quotes from nurses in our research study, in all positions of leadership, revealed the importance of self-awareness demonstrated through humility and the ability to recognize humanity in self and others. One nurse in the research study mentioned that a leader is *not always popular* but is self-assured and confident. The Upholder demonstrates self-management as they *adjust* and *support the team in stressful situations*. The leader as Upholder is socially and organizationally aware, being careful not to *play favorites* but instead *give everyone a fair chance*. When an Upholder is embedded within the team, the vision, work, and outcomes belong to the team rather than to the leader alone. Being socially and organizationally aware as an embedded leader is a hallmark of the Upholder. The Upholder is a liaison between potential competing priorities of upper leadership and the point-of-service priorities.

The Socially and Organizationally Aware Leader in Action

Jean Watson, theorist and expert in the "Art of Caring," suggests the following ways to demonstrate **"Caring in Action,"** which correlate with these attributes of the Upholder:

- Creating healing environments—attending to the subtle environment. For example, paying attention to details in the environment such as an uncluttered and organized nurse's station or patient rooms.
- Interviewing and selecting staff based on "caring" orientation. For example, asking candidates to describe a "Caring Moment."
- Making human caring integral to the organizational vision and culture. For example, integrate caring language into the vision, mission, and values statements.
- Placing reminders of caring practices in the environment. For example, place magnets on the patients' door with positive affirmations.
- Exploring the integration of caring language in documentation. For example, document "caring rounds."
- Displaying healing objects in accordance with patients' wishes; for example, prayer mats, crosses, stones, mandalas, and artwork (Watson, 2009).

Personally Well and Healthy

As you embody the traits of the Upholder, you will focus on personal resiliency and well-being, which are achieved through the practices discussed earlier: self-awareness, self-compassion, self-care, and mindfulness. Through modeling these "self" practices along with mindfulness, you will be better able to connect, care, and intentionally focus on others. In turn, the caregivers will appreciate the caring interactions and be influenced to assess and improve their own resiliency and wellness practices. As you model these practices, the team will realize the importance of prioritizing these habits in their own lives. Upholders can function as "point attractors," which Crowell (2016) describes as a pattern of behavior that attracts like behavior in a complex system. Through role-modeling wellness practices and demonstrating new ways of leading, the Upholder creates their own butterfly effect, meaning their seemingly small behaviors can have an enormous impact due to the sensitivity and interconnectivity of the staff and the structures within the organization.

Because of the nature of healthcare, the work environment in a unit needs to reflect care and caring. The team members want to feel comfortable, safe, and cared for, and

The Personally Well and Healthy Leader in Action

Watson (2009), theorist and expert in the "Art of Caring," suggests the following ways to demonstrate **"Caring in Action,"** which correlate with these attributes of the Upholder:

- Cultivating your own spiritual practices
- Cultivating heart-centered practices of loving kindness
- Cultivating self-control and calm in yourself and others
- Engaging in centering exercises
- Engaging in mindfulness practices
- Participating in multi-site research assessing caring among staff and patients
- Creating opportunities to share caring moments
- Creating innovative practice models or patterns around the delivery of care
- Developing "caring competencies" to guide caring practice. For example, using active listening with patients and colleagues, sitting at the bedside when possible, and including family in the conversation.

they want to know that they hold an important position within the organization. They want to feel that the work they're doing connects them to their purpose. While this can sound overwhelming for a leader, it's something that evolves as the culture changes, and over time a culture of caring develops. Nurses, as humans caring for other humans, must first show care for themselves and be cared for before they can do the same for others. We've all heard the phrase, "You can't give what you don't have." This simple wisdom explains why the work of the human-centered leader, acting as an Upholder, is so important. Care for the caregivers results in an improved experience for all.

As an Upholder, you embrace your own humanity and demonstrate self-compassion when mistakes are made. You'll want to be whole-hearted, and according to Brown (2010), that means inherently vulnerable. You are willing to take ownership of your mistakes and absorb criticisms. This is not the part of leadership that leaders enjoy thinking about. It does, however, reveal why leaders must be courageous to be authentic. The vulnerability and authenticity of a leader demonstrate strength rather than weakness and open the door for a strong connection and relationship with staff members.

The Upholder Meets Complexity

As a leader who embodies the Upholder attributes, embracing self-reflection and emotional awareness is essential. By practicing mindfulness with intention, you demonstrate to your team that you are fully present—whether in conversations with them, colleagues, or patients.

Because Human-Centered Leadership is built on relationships, the Upholder attributes create a strong foundation for authentic communication, openness, and the free flow of information. In a complex, adaptive system, your commitment to nonhierarchical communication fosters meaningful connections. These connections—both within your team and across disciplines—help spark self-organization, the breeding ground for innovation. Crowell (2016) said it well . . . the strength of a team's relationships directly impacts the quality of healthcare outcomes.

> The Upholder, who ensures that relationships are authentic, collaborative, and free from judgment, is the cornerstone on which self-organization, innovation, and positive outcomes develop.

Outcomes Resulting from a Culture of Caring

The culture of caring goes beyond impacting the team and patients on a personal level. It also impacts quality care and safe practice by fostering team behaviors and collaboration. When mistakes happen, team members speak up more comfortably, knowing that no one will blame or shame them, but that the team will support them and work to improve systems that will prevent the same mistake in the future. According to Watson (2007, 2009), a caring and supportive environment leads to a decrease in adverse events.

As you practice the attributes of the Upholder, your leadership skills will contribute to a culture of caring and your outcomes will align closely with those required by the American Nurses Credentialing Center (ANCC) Magnet Recognition Program standards (2023) and the ANCC Pathway to Excellence standards (2020).

The leader influences the Magnet Standards of Transformational Leadership, Structural Empowerment, Exemplary Professional Practice, and New Knowledge, Innovations and Improvements embracing the dimension of the Upholder. See Appendix E for examples. The ANCC Magnet Recognition Program requires empirical outcomes related to a culture of caring. These outcomes include decreased turnover rates, improved patient experience, greater responsiveness to patients' feedback (service recovery), and greater RN satisfaction, which includes access to leadership, the responsiveness of leaders, autonomy, interprofessional relationships, quality care, and adequate resources (ANCC, 2023; Appendix E).

The ANCC Pathway to Excellence Framework (2020) also includes standards that rely on a culture of caring. These standards include:

Pathway Standard 3 (Safety): Ensures that nurses' safety and well-being are safeguarded. A safe environment includes having measures to create a culture free of incivility, bullying, and violence. Interprofessional decision-making welcomes diverse thoughts and promotes an inclusive culture.

Pathway Standard 4 (Quality): Ensures that educational sessions that address respectful communication are offered.

Pathway Standard 5 (Well-Being): Ensures that leadership embraces a shared governance culture and creates an environment that supports workforce well-being. This includes role-modeling behaviors of self-care (Appendix F).

From Knowing to Doing: Practical Ways to Influence a Culture of Caring

To understand how the Upholder cultivates a culture of caring, we turn to the framework of *Being-Knowing-Doing*. When values, mindset, and knowledge come together, they create the foundation for meaningful action. This progression illustrates how the Upholder moves from Being (values and mindset) to Knowing (knowledge) to Doing (caring actions). Here are some practical ways to make the move from Knowing to Doing.

Model Care for Self

As a leader, your actions speak loudly and influence the behavior of the team. Realize the value of modeling care for your inner self to your team. Practice self-kindness, self-acceptance, and self-compassion. Commit to mindfulness practice, focusing on the importance of presence (Kabat-Zinn, 2023). Finally, prioritize your spirituality. Not only are these practices important for you personally, but also the impact on the team contributes to the culture of caring.

Rounding

Best practices encourage nurse leaders to round on staff routinely. This practice helps connect the staff member to the leader and helps to build trust, rapport, and demonstrate caring. Watson's (2009) theory reinforces the need for leaders to ensure that staff feel cared for, have the resources they need, and have the support of a collaborative team. To create a culture of caring, ask the staff member during leader–staff rounds:

1. Do you feel cared for on this unit?
2. What would make you feel more cared for?
3. Do you have the tools and equipment you need to care for your patients?
4. Do you have the support of the team to provide the best care to your patients?

Recognizing Supportive Team Members

You find that there are many ways to recognize your supportive team members. You'll need to determine which works best on your unit.

1. If you huddle during or at the end of the shift, ask if anyone can give a call out to a team member for supporting them in caring for a patient.
2. Keep notes on a bulletin board and encourage staff to write a short note about a team member who supported them during the shift and post it to the "TEAM" board.
3. What other ideas do you have? ______________________________

Encourage Reflection Among Team Members

Help staff understand the value of learning by reflecting on experience. You may refer them to "Shifts: The Journal for Nurses by Nurses" (2021). The journal provides an easy way to begin a reflective practice by organizing your thoughts and learnings in the SBAR format.

Make Self-Care and Work–Life Harmony a Priority for Yourself and Your Team Members

1. Ask team members what they are doing to take care of themselves. Make sure that the team is taking their lunch and dinner breaks, practicing mindful moments, using deep breathing for relaxing during breaks, and taking appropriate time off.
2. Encourage staff participation in wellness activities. One organization did a wellness challenge to see who could clock the most steps on their device over one month. The winner was recognized and received a membership at the organization's wellness center.
3. One CNO colleague does her one-on-one meetings with her directors as "walking" meetings as a way to promote wellness in self and others.
4. What other ideas do you have to prioritize well-being with your team?

Discussion Questions for Groups

1. What are the metrics you currently follow to ensure a culture of caring?
2. What additional metrics could you consider to facilitate an environment where staff are satisfied and experience meaningful work and patients report positive experiences (refer to Table 3)?
3. As a leader, develop S.M.A.R.T. goals to improve your practice of the Upholder attributes. Include goals around the following: personal wellness,

self-awareness, mindfulness, others-oriented mindset, and social and organizational awareness. Discuss your goals with your colleagues. How will you work together and harness the wisdom of the team? How can you help each other?

4. How can you infuse the environment with the expectation of positive staff interrelationships and caring service to your patients?
5. What resources do you have available to you to promote wellness, mindfulness, and positive relationships among your staff? What else is needed?

Reflection Questions for Individuals

Have you ever experienced a culture of caring? If this is your current experience, how will you continue to nurture and protect this culture? If this is not your current experience, how can you begin to impact the culture through care for yourself, your staff, and your patients?

____

____

____

____

____

References

American Nurses Credentialing Center. (2023). *Magnet application manual.* ANCC.

Bradberry, T., & Greaves, J. (2009). *Emotional intelligence 2.0.* TalentSmart.

Brown, B. (2010). *The gifts of imperfection: Let go of who you think you're supposed to be and embrace who you are.* Hazelden.

Brown, B. (2018, October 15). *Clear is kind. Unclear is unkind.* Retrieved from https://brenebrown.com/blog/2018/10/15/clear-is-kind-unclear-is-unkind

Chang, D. F., Donald, J., Whitney, J., Miao, I. Y., & Sahdra, B. (2024). Does Mindfulness Improve Intergroup Bias, Internalized Bias, and Anti-Bias Outcomes?: A Meta-Analysis of the Evidence and Agenda for Future Research. *Personality & social psychology bulletin, 50*(10), 1487–1516. doi: 10.1177/01461672231178518

Crowell, D. M. (2016). *Complexity leadership* (2nd ed.). FA Davis Co.

Fulford, M. D., & Coleman, R. A. (2021). Maximizing the value of values-based leadership (VBL): A reconceptualization for leaders and organizations. *Journal of Applied Leadership and Management, 9*, 61–72. Retrieved from https://journal-alm.org/article/view/22350/14336

Goleman, D., Boyatzis, R., & McKee, A. (2013). *Primal leadership: Unleashing the power of emotional intelligence.* Harvard Business Review Press.

Hernandez, M. & Summers, C. (2024, April 25). Effective leaders articulate values - and live by them. *MIT Sloan Management Review.* Retrieved from https://sloanreview.mit.edu/article/effective-leaders-articulate-values-and-live-by-them/

Hougaard, R., Carter, J., & Hobson, N. (2020, December 4). *Leadership & managing people. Compassionate leadership is necessary—but not sufficient.* Harvard Business Review. Retrieved from https://hbr.org/2020/12/compassionate-leadership-is-necessary-but-not-sufficient

Kabat-Zinn, J. (2023). Mindfulness-based interventions in context: Past, present, and future. *Clinical Psychology, 10*(2), 144–156. Retrieved from https://jonkabat-zinn.com/wp-content/uploads/2023/01/JonKabat-Zinn_MindfulnessBased-InterventionsContext.pdf

Leclerc, L., Kennedy, K., & Campis, S. (2021). Human-centered leadership in healthcare: A contemporary nursing leadership theory generated via constructivist grounded theory. *Journal of Nursing Management, 29*(2), 294–306.

Watson, J. (2007). Caring theory as an ethical guide to administrative and clinical practices. *Nursing Administration Quarterly, 30*(1), 48–55.

Watson, J. (2009). Caring science and human caring theory: Transforming personal and professional practices of nursing and health care. *Journal of Health and Human Services Administration, 31*(4), 466–482.

Recommended Reading

Goulston, M., & Hendel, D. (2020). *Why cope when you can heal? How healthcare heroes of Covid-19 can recover from PTSD.* Harper Horizon.

Graham, L. (2013). *Bouncing back: Rewiring your brain for maximum resilience and well-being.* New World Library.

Grant, A. (2023). *Hidden potential: The science of achieving greater things.* Viking.

Kennedy, K., Leclerc, L., & Campis, S. (2021). *Shifts: The journal for nurses by nurses.* Morgan James Publishing.

Leclerc, L., & Pabico, C. (2023). A blueprint for well-being: Modeling the way through Human-Centered Leadership and Pathway to Excellence. *Nursing Management, 54*(4), 9–16. doi: 10.1097/01.NUMA.0000921892.27917.78

Steidle, G. K. (2018). *Leading from within: Conscious social change and mindfulness for social innovation.* MIT Press.

CHAPTER 10

Real People, Real Results!

A weak leader likes to tell us how many people work for them. A great leader is humbled to tell us how many people they work for.

—Simon Sinek, Author and inspirational speaker

Human-Centered Leadership in Healthcare (HCL-HC) continues to make a meaningful impact, reaching nurses and leaders across both academic and clinical settings. In this chapter, we share stories from academia, DNP students who have applied this model to their scholarly projects, and healthcare leaders who have embraced and implemented HCL-HC in their organizations. Some organizations have implemented Human-Centered Leadership (HCL) across their entire institution, while others have introduced it within specific departments of larger systems. Regardless of the scope, when the leadership team actively supports and embraces this model, the impact is profound—strengthening outcomes for leaders, staff, and patients alike.

The Value of a Framework: Human-Centered Leadership in Healthcare

By Bradly Phillips, Chief Nurse Anesthetist, Vice Chair of Advanced Practice and Allied Health Professions, MD Anderson Cancer Center

As the healthcare leader and Chief Nurse Anesthetist at a large tertiary specialty hospital, I found myself drawn to the HCL-HC model through my experiences with the Coldiron Senior Nurse Executive program at Case Western Reserve University. This framework resonated deeply with my personal leadership style and provided the structure needed to elevate my approach.

Recognizing its potential, I introduced the framework to the leaders on my team. Together, we embraced HCL-HC as our guiding compass for fostering meaningful connections, empowering our team, and achieving exceptional results.

As a leader, I place high value on creating a culture built on psychological safety, just culture principles, and high reliability. I consider emotional intelligence to be an integral part of everyday leadership practice. While our organization offers well-developed programs supporting these concepts, the HCL-HC framework adds an underpinning structure that uniquely bridges daily practices and team member responses, co-creating a culture that drives sustainable outcomes.

Since adopting the framework, we have recognized our recent, ongoing, and future leadership initiatives that model HCL-HC. For example, we had certified registered nurse anesthetist (CRNA) leadership-led High Reliability Training delivered to our CRNA team, integrated safety and recognition moments in all our staff meetings, and implemented a just-culture framework. We also revamped the structure of our one-on-one meetings to prioritize the whole person, ensuring our conversations go beyond tasks to address individual needs. We shifted our scheduling process, offering greater flexibility and alternative shifts tailored to team members' preferences. To further promote well-being, our Assistant Chief CRNA and CRNA manager wellness champions introduced maternity scrubs for pregnant team members—a thoughtful touch that reflects our commitment to care and inclusiveness.

Our focus on cultivating a team culture rooted in safety, relationships, and well-being has yielded remarkable results. In our most recent engagement survey, we achieved a participation rate of 91%, with an overall engagement score of 92.

This shared mental model of HCL-HC connects the dots for leaders from their values and behaviors to the culture they create and the results they influence. It provides alignment, structure, and guidance for the team. Our success in improving our team culture continues to be recognized by our department, division, and across the organization.

From Vision to Reality: Transforming Leadership Culture at UCLA Health

By Jessica Phillips, Executive Director, Nursing Practice, Education, and Research, UCLA Health

I worked with the uLeadership team to spearhead the transformative implementation of the HCL-HC model across the health system. Beginning in April 2023, the professional development team leaders and a group of 200 nurse leaders embarked on an ambitious journey to embed HCL-HC principles into organizational culture through the Human-Centered Leadership in Healthcare Essentials program.

The initiative kicked off with an on-site introduction to HCL-HC and an appreciative inquiry focused on wellness, growth, and retention. The team asked leaders to reflect on past successes and strengths, exploring what has worked well and what currently thrives within the organization. Building on this foundation, the team then transitioned to the "dream" phase, envisioning ideal future scenarios and answering the profound question: "What do wellness, growth, and retention ideally look like?"

To ensure a seamless and meaningful integration, UCLA's Professional Development leaders coordinated participation in uLeadership's *Human-Centered Leadership in Healthcare Essentials* program, incorporating self-reflection exercises and a book study. Their goal was clear: to foster genuine cultural change, embedding HCL-HC into the fabric of the organization rather than treating it as a one-off professional development initiative.

A critical element of the effort was aligning the dimensions of HCL-HC with the Mission, Vision, and Values of UCLA Health. This integration also included mapping HCL-HC against Relationship-Based Care®—an established model for transforming practice at the bedside. The shared tenets underscored the harmony between HCL-HC and UCLA Health's existing care delivery framework.

Postimplementation, HCL-HC principles became foundational across various organizational programs and structures. They incorporated the theory into Nursing Orientation; Preceptor Development Training; and Research, Evidence-Based Practice, and Innovation initiatives. Additionally, HCL-HC influenced the Professional

Governance structure, guiding training for chairs and co-chairs. It became integral to the Transition to Practice programs for both new graduates and new leaders, as well as the organization's mentoring program.

As the cultural shift takes hold, UCLA Health is exploring its outcomes. A longitudinal research study is currently underway, assessing qualitative insights from the appreciative inquiry process and quantitative results from surveys on well-being, growth, and retention. While the study spans one year postimplementation, preliminary results already suggest HCL-HC has cemented its position as a cornerstone of leadership culture.

Today, HCL-HC is viewed not as an initiative but as "the way things are done" in an organization driven by compassion, excellence, discovery, integrity, teamwork, and equity. UCLA Health continues to inspire, innovate, and lead the charge for HCL-HC.

Human-Centered Leadership in Healthcare: The Foundation to the Execution of a Nursing Strategic Plan

By Karen Steiner, Retired System Director, Nursing Professional Practice, Summa Health

Penelope Gorsuch, Senior Vice President and Chief Nurse Executive, Summa Health

Karrie Boss, System Director Evidence-Based Practice, Summa Health

Bonnie Jensen, Vice President, Chief Nursing Officer, Summa Health

Imagine a healthcare system where the nursing staff had input into strategic initiatives and nurse leaders were equipped with a skillset to drive implementation and change that not only delivered exceptional patient care but also drove a $44 million financial impact. This is the result at Akron, Ohio-based Summa Health following the implementation of a comprehensive nursing strategic plan and the adoption of the HCL-HC framework. Nursing's vision was to elevate our practice and improve patient, clinician, and organizational outcomes. However, the team could not have been accomplished without the implementation of a nursing leadership framework specifically developed to guide the leader in cultivating a culture of caring, trust, and excellence.

The four priorities for nursing included all-inclusive organizational care, interprofessional collaborative care, person-centered precision care, and patients' and healthcare professionals' self-care. They executed goals through a two-year phased approach, ensuring focus on the measurable outcomes that directly impacted the organization's financial performance.

Significant goals included:

1. Creation of the Center for Clinical Inquiry®, a dual operating system to promote and support change
2. Leadership development to implement change
3. Restructuring of the hospital nursing department based on the span of control
4. Redesign and implementation of an evidence-based nursing professional governance structure

One hundred two nurse leaders at Summa Health participated in HCL-HC training. The participants included nurse leaders from the Human Resources Professional Development Department, nurse managers, nursing directors, associate chief nursing officers, chief nursing officer, chief nurse executive, nursing system directors, clinical nurse specialists, and nurse educators, from acute care and ambulatory settings.

The training consisted of the Human-Centered Leadership in Healthcare Essentials course, which contains five modules, each two hours in length. Each participant received a copy of the *Human-Centered Leadership in Healthcare* book and was asked to participate in a book study with their peers to discuss the application of HCL-HC in their daily practice.

They held the educational sessions on Microsoft Teams once per month from January through May and recorded them, so those unable to attend the live session could participate. In addition to the monthly modules, they held six optional book club sessions on Microsoft Teams for all participating leaders. The purpose of these sessions was to foster further discussion and reflection on information learned in the modules and from within the book.

Providing nurse leaders with a healthcare leadership framework developed by nurses for nurses has made an impact. Nurse leader engagement scores have remained consistently high from 2023 to 2025, with a statistically significant improvement in leader mindfulness eight months after the training concluded.

One of the outcomes related to our strategic plan was the creation of the Center for Clinical Inquiry. The Center for Clinical Inquiry Model incorporates an evidence-based decision-making process with the dimensions of HCL-HC. This approach promotes and supports staff in delivering the best care by creating a culture of caring, trust, and excellence, which is the essential foundation of HCL-HC (Figure 7).

Creating these measurable goals led to a cultural change that provided clear direction and purpose, which aligned individual and organizational actions with shared values. Our nurses gained a new sense of focus and motivation, supporting and encouraging them to adopt new behaviors and best practices that elevated the practice of nursing. Additionally, these measurable goals allowed our progress to be tracked; reinforced our commitment to change; and created a culture of competence, compassion, accountability, and trust.

Significant outcomes included:

1. First-year nurse turnover rate decreased from 26% in 2022 to 13% in 2024.
2. Overall nursing turnover rate decreased from 19% in 2022 to 12% in 2024, saving approximately $9.4 million.

FIGURE 7
Professional Practice Model implemented at the Center for Clinical Inquiry at Summa Health.

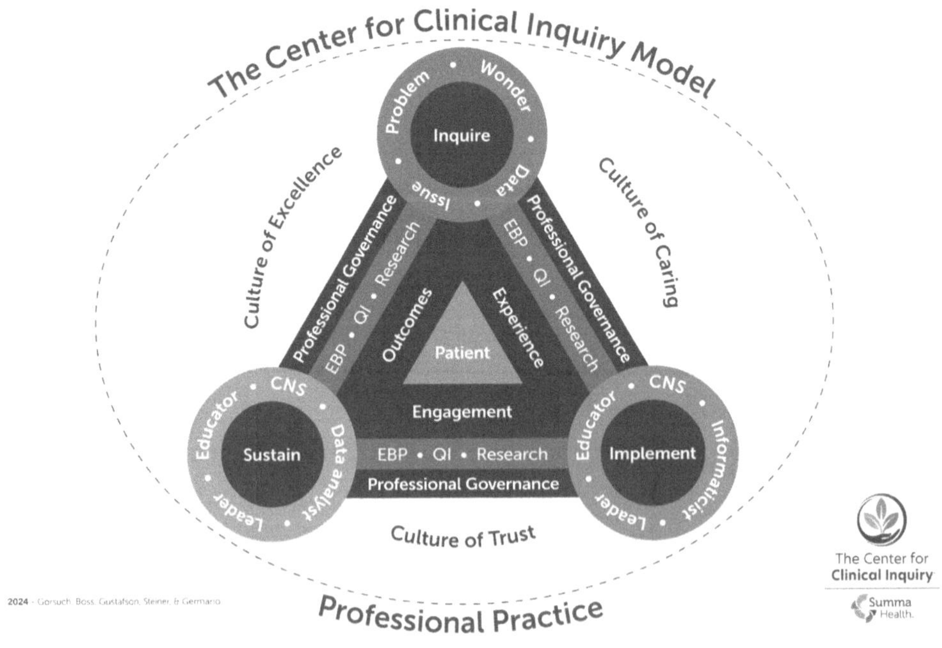

3. Zero nurse leader turnover from 2023 through the first quarter of 2025.
4. Agency spend decreased by $22 million from 2022 to 2024.
5. Nine evidence-based practice initiatives were implemented over two years, which demonstrated a $6.8 million cost avoidance.

By aligning nursing strategic initiatives with the HCL-HC framework and using a systematic approach to drive change, our nurses are pivotal in achieving patient, clinician, and organizational outcomes. Creating a focus on building leaders while supporting and elevating nursing practice has resulted in a significant impact on our organization and the community we serve.

Inclusive Excellence: A Human-Centered Approach to Thriving

By Katie Boston-Leary, PhD, MBA, MHA, RN, NEA-BC, FAONL, FADLN, FAAN Senior Vice President of Equity and Engagement, American Nurses Enterprise

G. Rumay Alexander, Ed.D, MSN, BSN, RN, FAAN, FADLN, Senior Equity Advisor, American Nurses Association, Professor, School of Nursing, The University of North Carolina at Chapel Hill

In the heart of a fast-paced metropolitan academic hospital, a new kind of leadership conversation was taking place. Over two transformative days, a powerful collaboration between uLeadership and the American Nurses Association, led by Katie Boston-Leary and G. Rumay Alexander, brought healthcare leaders together for an experience titled *Cultural Fluency to Thrive: Leadership for the Modern Era.*

It wasn't just another training. It was a mindset shift.

Katie and Rumay brought deep expertise in integrating Diversity, Equity, Inclusion, and Belonging (DEIB) principles—essential elements supported by the HCL-HC framework. Specifically, they shared a relatable correlation between Maslow's Hierarchy of Needs and the components of DEIB, ultimately leading to *Human Flourishing* and resulting in *Inclusive Excellence* (Boston-Leary, Alexander, & Davis, 2024). Their guidance helped participants move beyond theory and into practice, showing that embracing our shared humanity is key to leading with intention and impact.

As healthcare teams face the constant pressures of a VUCA world—volatile, uncertain, complex, and ambiguous—the session introduced a fresh response: a leadership approach rooted in empathy, equity, and belonging. At the center of it, all were DEIB principles, not as buzzwords, but as foundational strategies for leading with purpose and impact.

Participants leaned into honest conversations about trust, authenticity, and inclusion. They unpacked complex topics such as oppression, meritocracy, and colorism—not with blame or defensiveness, but with openness and courage. Through reflective exercises and powerful storytelling, they walked away with tools to lead in ways that make others feel genuinely seen, respected, and valued.

And the feedback? It was overwhelmingly positive!

Hospital leaders described the session as timely, relevant, and deeply necessary. Many felt it gave them fresh language and clarity to face complexity with confidence. With the shared mental model of HCL as their compass, they returned to their teams ready to lead not just with strategic intent—but with heart.

This wasn't just a workshop. It was the beginning of a movement—toward leadership that recognizes humanity as its greatest strength.

Reference

Boston-Leary, K., Alexander, G. R., & Davis, S. (2024). Leveraging Maslow's hierarchy of needs to build nursing's more inclusive future. *Nursing Administration Quarterly, 48*(1), 55–64.

Results Through Relationships: A Human-Centered Leadership Success Story

By Kassandra Meadows, Administrative Director, Perinatal Services, Christus Children's

As an experienced leader starting an interim assignment at HCA Clearlake Medical Center in Webster, Texas, I stepped into a position with a challenging mission ahead. Upon entering the department, I immediately observed the impact of low morale and leader burnout. The metrics confirmed these initial observations, with turnover rates hovering around 30%—month over month. I knew I had to take decisive action to turn the situation around.

My introduction to HCL-HC came serendipitously through listening to a podcast with the uLeadership team and reading the book, *Human-Centered Leadership in*

Healthcare: Evolution of a Revolution. Inspired by the principles in this book, I shared them with the team, and we moved toward implementation of the model within the department. With a core group of eight leaders, the team began its journey toward redefining what leadership looked like.

The leadership team began to prioritize self-care and strengthened their focus on reward and meaningful recognition of their staff. The implementation period lasted around four months. Within this remarkably short period, the staff turnover rate dropped to 0%. This improvement was sustained over the next year, with turnover stabilizing between 2.1% and 2.6%.

Employee engagement saw equally significant results. Participation in the employee engagement survey rose from 12% to 61%, and overall engagement scores climbed from 56 to 76. Results demonstrated agreement with key statements such as "My manager recognizes me as a person," which increased by 17 points, and agreement with statements on reward and recognition, which soared by 26 points.

The ripple effects extended beyond staff engagement. The patient experience scores, which had previously hovered around the 51st percentile, skyrocketed to the 97th percentile within just four months of implementing the model.

Checking back with this leadership team, one year postimplementation of HCL-HC, they shared that they have not lost a single leader. The staff turnover continued to remain below 5%. And the patient experience scores remain at the 97th percentile.

This work exemplifies the impact that HCL-HC can make on a leadership team and the impact the engaged, relationship-focused leaders then make with their team members, patients, and culture. It's true that you do get results through relationships. It starts with you, but it's not *about* you!

Healing Through Leadership: UH Ahuja Medical Center's Cultural Transformation

By Stephanie Lonzo, Director of Critical Care, UH Ahuja Medical Center

Lindsey Colangelo, Chief Nursing Officer, UH Ahuja Medical Center

In early 2023, UH Ahuja Medical Center, part of University Hospitals in Cleveland, Ohio, embarked on a bold HCL-HC initiative to address mounting challenges. Severe staffing shortages, cultural fragmentation, and the complexities of doubling hospital capacity following a multimillion-dollar expansion created a critical need for change. The executive leaders within the organization sought to rebuild engagement and teamwork in the postpandemic era through a unifying cultural reset.

Stephanie and Lindsey collaborated with the uLeadership team to implement a systemwide engagement and leadership development program. This initiative included an on-site introduction to HCL-HC, an appreciative inquiry exercise on values and identity, virtual interactive Learning Labs, cross-departmental book clubs, and self-reflection exercises. The team also developed a unifying mission, "Be the Best Ahuja," and introduced their daily guiding values. These elements were designed to foster connection and purpose across teams.

Change was embedded at the frontline level through customized departmental action plans, daily huddles, and progress tracking using clear Objectives and Key Results. Staff added personal touches, such as displaying their "why" for working in healthcare on badge backers, cultivating resilience, and grounding them in their purpose.

The outcomes of this initiative led to profound and meaningful changes. Workforce turnover improved significantly, with RN turnover dropping from 27.29% to 19.61% and first-year RN turnover decreasing from 60% to 28%. Remarkably, nursing leadership turnover reached 0%, and non-clinical departments experienced minimal turnover. Patient experience surveys revealed gains across all categories, with inpatient scores showing substantial improvement. Accountability culture strengthened, engagement among nurse managers soared to 93%, and staff-driven initiatives created a strong sense of ownership.

Quality outcomes saw remarkable progress as well. Targeted areas maintained zero catheter-associated urinary tract infections or central line-associated bloodstream infections for over a year, falls were reduced through frontline-led initiatives, and departments took pride in shaping their own quality improvement processes. Cultural shifts included the introduction of activities such as Wellness Wednesdays, a transition from Nurses Week to an inclusive Hospital Week, and collaborative goal setting between staff and managers. Leadership development played a pivotal role in sustainability, with emerging leaders gaining critical management skills and nurse managers achieving certifications.

Throughout this journey, the organization observed key lessons. The steadfast commitment of leadership, cross-role relationship building, and recognition of every team member's value proved to be the foundation of success. By modeling well-being, fostering trust, and empowering teams, UH Ahuja Medical Center demonstrated the profound impact of HCL-HC on transforming culture and enhancing patient care.

Leading with Humanity: Strengthening Nurse Leadership Through Human-Centered Preceptorship

By Adam Meier, Chief Nursing Officer, University of Kansas Health System. Project completed at the University of Kansas Health System, Kansas City Campus, as part of a Doctor of Nursing Practice Program at the University of Missouri, Sinclair School of Nursing.

The HCL-HC framework served as the foundation for a pilot program designed to strengthen preceptorship for nurse leaders in preceptor roles. The leadership preceptor plays a crucial role in shaping the success of new nurse managers—enhancing their preparedness, effectiveness, and long-term retention.

This program focuses on a leader's ability to serve as a Connector, Awakener, and Upholder, aligning closely with the essential qualities needed for impactful nursing leadership. By integrating the HCL-HC framework, the preceptor program not only addresses the technical aspects of leadership but also the human elements essential for fostering trust, excellence, and compassionate care (Kennedy, Leclerc, & Campis, 2021).

The quality improvement project took place at the University of Kansas Health System, Kansas City Campus, as part of a Doctor of Nursing Practice Project at the University of Missouri, Sinclair School of Nursing. The curriculum was intentionally designed with the HCL-HC model in mind, ensuring preceptors could take a learner-centered approach, adapt to different learning modalities, provide constructive feedback, and effectively evaluate performance.

To measure the impact of the program, three assessment tools evaluated preceptors' commitment, confidence, and competence in mentoring new nurse leaders: the Commitment to the Preceptor Role and Preceptor's Perception of Support Tools (Diber & Goldenberg, 1995), the Preceptor Self-Assessment Tool (Guthrie et al., 2023), and the Modified Capstone Experience Preceptor Preparedness Scale (L'Ecuyer et al., 2022).

The project aimed for a 5% increase in median scores across all three domains, but the results exceeded expectations—showing an 8% increase, with statistically significant improvements in enjoyment, confidence, and competence.

These findings underscore the importance of strengthening leadership preceptors in nursing. A well-supported onboarding and transition process ensures that new nurse leaders enter their roles with the skills and confidence they need. Ultimately, HCL-HC is key to building a strong professional community, cultivating trust, and recognizing the humanity in those learning to lead. By embracing this model, healthcare organizations can create stability, sustainability, and a thriving leadership culture.

References

Diber, C., & Goldenberg, D. (1995). Preceptor's perceptions of benefits, rewards, supports, and commitment to the preceptor role. *Journal of Advanced Nursing, 21*(6), 1144–1151.

Guthrie, L. E., Marszalek, J., & Lasiter, S. (2023). Psychometric testing of a scale measuring preceptor preparedness: The Cap-ExPres™ study. *Journal of Nursing Measurement, 31*(3), 325–335. doi: 10.1891/JNM-2022-0023

Kennedy, K., Leclerc, L., & Campis, S. (2021). *Human-Centered Leadership in Healthcare: Evolution of a Revolution.* Morgan James Publishing.

L'Ecuyer, K., Subramaniam, D., Reangsing, C., & DuBois, J. (2022). Psychometric testing of the Preceptor Self-Assessment Tool (PSAT)-40 for nursing preceptors. *Journal of Continuing Education in Nursing, 53*(11), 491–499. doi: 10.3928/00220124-20221006-06

Reimagining Joy in Work: Nurse Managers in the Inpatient Setting

By Daniel Ramberger, Chief Nursing Officer, Kaiser Permanente-Redwood City. Project completed at Stanford Health Care as part of the Doctor of Nursing Practice program at the University of California San Francisco.

Burnout and declining engagement among nurse managers are pressing challenges in healthcare. To combat this, the "Reimagining Joy in Work" initiative was launched at a large academic medical center in Northern California. The project aimed to restore a sense of purpose and connection for 40 inpatient nurse managers, with the support of eight operational directors and executive nursing leadership.

The program introduced three key strategies to foster engagement:

1. **Weekly in-person team meetings** led by operational directors to build camaraderie and alignment.
2. **Shared team meals** to encourage informal, personal connections.
3. **Weekly wellness walks** focused on gratitude, self-care, and unplugging from daily stress.

Additionally, an optional book club featuring *Human-Centered Leadership in Healthcare: Evolution of a Revolution* provided intellectual inspiration and learning opportunities.

Despite holiday disruptions, overall participation was strong, and the results were promising. After the 10-week program, participants reported an increase in joy and meaning in their work, as measured by the *Meaning and Joy in Work Questionnaire* (Rutledge, Wickman, & Winokur, 2018). Five individual questionnaire items showed statistically significant improvement ($p < 0.05$), particularly those related to dignity and respect, feeling valued, energy from positive experiences, spiritual well-being, and alignment with personal goals. The cumulative engagement score for the project participants increased by 6.18% over this time frame.

The program's low-cost, relationship-centered approach provided a meaningful step toward improving nurse manager well-being and engagement—an outcome essential for retention and leadership success in complex healthcare environments.

References

Rutledge, D. N., Wickman, M., & Winokur, E. J. (2018). Instrument validation: Hospital nurse perceptions of meaning and joy in work. *Journal of Nursing Measurement, 26*(3), 579–588. doi: 10.1891/1061-3749.26.3.579

Human-Centered Leadership in Healthcare: Impact on Mindfulness Practice Among Nurse Leaders

By Karen Steiner, Retired System Director, Nursing Professional Practice, Summa Health. Project completed at Summa Health as part of a Doctor of Nursing Practice program at the Frances Payne Bolton School of Nursing at Case Western Reserve University.

As a hospital leader for over 20 years, I have witnessed the challenges of sustaining quality leadership and resilient teams. The HCL-HC framework profoundly influenced my perspective, emphasizing relational leadership rooted in self-compassion, self-awareness, and mindfulness. These principles inspired my Doctor of Nursing Practice (DNP) scholarly project while attending the Frances Payne Bolton School of Nursing at Case Western Reserve. The project evaluated the impact of HCL-HC adoption on nurse leader mindfulness and engagement within a 1,027-bed nonprofit, Magnet-designated hospital system in Northeast Ohio.

The findings were illuminating. Mindfulness levels among nurse leaders improved after the intervention to the level of statistical significance, demonstrating the framework's value in fostering awareness and resilience. Demographic factors such as leadership experience and professional certification did not significantly impact mindfulness scores, though slightly higher scores were observed among those with nursing certifications. Engagement levels remained stable, with no significant differences between pre- and postintervention scores. Interestingly, engagement scores were strong before the implementation and remained strong postintervention, even though the organization underwent an acquisition during the same time frame.

While engagement outcomes did not shift measurably, this journey reinforced the transformative power of HCL-HC in nurturing mindfulness and fostering relational connections. For me, this framework is more than a leadership method—it's a revolutionary approach to leading, connecting, and inspiring within healthcare.

Transforming Leadership from Within: The Augusta University College of Nursing Journey

By Bill Hamilton, Assistant Dean and Associate Professor, Augusta University College of Nursing

I have spent the last three years embedding the principles of HCL-HC into a required DNP leadership course, offered twice a year. His mission is clear: to shape doctoral-prepared nurses not only as effective leaders but also as resilient, reflective, and compassionate individuals.

The course welcomes students from diverse specialties—acute care, pediatrics, psychiatric-mental health, family nurse practitioners, and nurse anesthetists—all at pivotal moments in their careers. These are seasoned professionals and practicing nurses seeking to elevate their leadership skills, and this course offers something unconventional: a deep dive into the idea that "self" is the foundation for leadership.

A cornerstone of the module was a simple breathing mindfulness practice, which I introduced, paired with critical self-reflection exercises. Students began by completing a Perceived Stress Scale survey (Cohen, Kamarck, & Mermelstein, 1983), which has often revealed eye-opening insights into the toll of healthcare leaders' demanding roles. Over 14 days, they commit to daily meditation, setting aside moments of stillness amid their fast-paced lives. After completing the practice, the students retake the Perceived Stress Scale and conduct video critical reflections on their experience.

Additionally, the course requires students to identify leaders within their organization who embody the dimensions of HCL-HC: the Awakener, the Connector, and the Upholder. Through these exercises, they link leadership theory to real-world examples, critically reflecting on how these dimensions align with or diverge from the HCL-HC model. This experience-based learning exercise supports the course's theoretical framework of adult learning, as espoused by Knowles (1984), linking the relevance of subject matter and learning activities to localized job or personal situations.

I noticed a profound ripple effect among the students. Across the cohort, students began to express renewed enthusiasm for their roles. The integration of the American Association of Critical Care Nurses Essential #10 into the program reinforced a culture of excellence, trust, and caring. The students, who were practicing nurses, reported feeling more equipped to lead with emotional intelligence—a skill often overlooked but essential for fostering cohesive teams.

The impact of the course was evident in the evaluations. Students consistently described it as impactful, practical, and life changing. Many highlighted the value of self-reflection and meditation, noting how these tools not only improved their leadership capabilities but also their overall well-being. A high focus on critical reflection—cognitive, affective, and process-oriented—ensured that the lessons extended far beyond the classroom.

Over 30 years, more than 350 students have passed through this leadership course. The feedback has been overwhelmingly positive: Students frequently mention how the course reshaped their approach to leadership, practice, and their DNP journey.

For me, the success of the program lies in its core message: "You cannot lead others until you can lead yourself." By instilling this philosophy in my students, I have not only enhanced their professional growth but also contributed to a more compassionate, effective healthcare system.

References

Cohen, S., Kamarck, T., & Mermelstein, R. (1983). A global measure of perceived stress. *Journal of Health and Social Behavior, 24*, 386–339. http://doi.org/10.2307/2136404

Knowles, M. (1984). *Andragogy in action.* Jossey-Bass.

Empowering Future Leaders: Human-Centered Leadership in Education

By Margie Sipe, Assistant Dean, Leadership Programs, Director, DNP Program, Associate Professor, MGH Institute of Healthcare Professions.

In an innovative partnership, uLeadership, LLC collaborated with the MGH Institute of Health Professions to introduce the HCL-HC framework into their DNP curriculum. This collaboration highlights the importance of preparing future leaders with the values and contemporary strategies needed to address the challenges of modern healthcare leadership.

The HCL-HC framework is presented to every DNP cohort, ensuring its principles are accessible to students during their postgraduate program for executive leaders and clinical leaders. Through engaging discussions and presentations, students learn how the model can be applied in real-world practice. This provides them with a clear pathway to connect theory with impactful action, whether in patient care, team management, or organizational transformation.

MGH Institute of Health Professions actively supports students in incorporating the HCL-HC framework into their DNP scholarly projects. For those interested in exploring this approach, the framework becomes a central component of their academic and professional journey. Using HCL principles in the implementation of their improvement projects enables students to support their colleagues and elevates their ability to deliver interventions that drive sustainable outcomes for patients. Additionally, by awakening, connecting, and upholding staff, leaders foster well-being and individual growth, supporting healthy work environments. This integration not only strengthens their theoretical foundation but also equips them to lead with empathy, purpose, and effectiveness.

Two notable recent projects exemplify these successes. The first project, "Restoring Joy to Nurse Leaders," by Dr. Jennifer Mills-Tamasi, focused on reducing burnout and stress while improving resilience and joy through mindfulness activities. Conducted at a 900-bed academic medical center, 13 nurse directors participated in weekly 30-minute sessions during their workday. These sessions included reflective writing, meditation, laughter yoga, and gratitude practices like "3 Good Things," facilitated by experts. Using the HCL-HC framework, this longitudinal study revealed a significant decrease in perceived stress and burnout among participants, highlighting the value of organizational support for mindfulness.

The second project, "Nurse Manager Stay Interview Training," by Dr. Linda Valentino, aimed to equip nurse managers with the skills to conduct stay interviews with their RN direct reports. This mixed-methods study involved 15 nurse leaders, who collectively conducted 246 interviews across 19 clinical units. Supported by the others-oriented attributes of the HCL-HC framework, the study proved the feasibility of training nurse managers in this strategy. Ultimately, it led to the broader implementation of stay interviews within the organization, strengthening retention efforts and fostering direct communication between leadership and staff. These initiatives underscore the impactful application of HCL-HC in addressing critical issues within healthcare leadership.

The collaboration has shown promising results, fostering a shared commitment to developing leaders who value connection, emotional intelligence, and relational strategies. The way we go about our work and strive to implement innovative solutions requires a strong focus on human-centered approaches. The integration of HCL-HC into academic curricula ensures that the next generation of healthcare professionals is equipped with tools to create cultures that prioritize well-being and achieve lasting results. By bridging academic learning with practical application, this partnership underscores the powerful potential of HCL-HC in shaping healthcare education and practice.

In Conclusion

It's been inspiring to share these real-world stories of growth, results, and success. We're grateful for the leaders who have poured their energy into becoming better and driving real change. The leaders featured here have embraced HCL-HC with passion and purpose, proving that meaningful change isn't just possible—it's happening. Their dedication is shaping academia and workplaces where teams thrive, patients receive better care, and safety and quality are more than just goals; they're lived experiences. And the most exciting part? This movement is only gaining momentum. The best is yet to come.

Discussion Questions for Groups

1. Reflecting on the stories shared in this chapter, which example of HCL-HC resonated most with you? How did leadership behaviors contribute to improved nurse retention, engagement, or patient experience, and what insights can be applied to your own practice?
2. The stories in this chapter illustrate both challenges and successes in implementing HCL-HC. What strategies or leadership approaches stood out as particularly effective? How can these lessons inform efforts to foster a more supportive and engaged nursing workforce in your own organization?

Reflection Questions for Individuals

1. Consider a time when you experienced or observed the principles of HCL-HC in action. How did it affect your sense of engagement, professional growth, or patient care? What aspects from the stories in this chapter align with or challenge your own experiences?

____

____

____

____

____

PART IV

Shaping a Culture Where People Flourish

To be effective, human-centered leaders must intentionally cultivate skills that enable them to foster a lasting culture of Well-Being, Excellence, Trust, and Caring. This development is crucial for creating an environment where team members feel valued, understood, and connected. These skills encompass Human-Centered Communication, Design, Understanding, and Belonging, fostering an environment where every team member feels valued and heard. Although not an exhaustive account, these essential skills are discussed in the following chapters.

Human-Centered Communication

Human-Centered Communication emphasizes the power of connection, inclusivity, and transformation in leadership. *Cultural intelligence* equips leaders to bridge differences, fostering collaboration and innovation by navigating diverse perspectives with respect and understanding. *Affirmative disruption* challenges outdated norms with optimism, replacing inertia with purposeful change and encouraging transparent, forward-thinking communication. Together with Human-Centered Leadership in Healthcare, these principles create an environment where dialogue fuels growth, trust, and meaningful progress in healthcare leadership.

CHAPTER 11

Cultural Intelligence

Fostering Meaningful Communication Through Human Connection

Every human is like all other humans, some other humans, and no other human.

—Clyde Kluckhon, American anthropologist

In today's world, where cultures are more intertwined than ever, cultural intelligence—often called cultural quotient (CQ)—has become an essential skill. You've probably heard the phrase "everything local is global," and it really captures how connected we all are. What happens in one community can ripple across the globe, while global trends shape the realities of everyday life.

Think about it—local cultures reflect the rich diversity of the world. No matter where you go, you're part of a global village, and this is especially clear in healthcare. In hospitals and clinics, professionals work alongside colleagues from all kinds of backgrounds, caring for patients whose cultural experiences span continents. It's a dynamic, deeply human exchange.

At its core, CQ is about the ability to adapt—whether it's in communication, behavior, or decision-making—so that interactions respect and reflect cultural differences. Whether you're part of an international team, working with clients from different backgrounds, or leading a diverse community, CQ helps you bridge gaps and build real connections. And in a world that increasingly values inclusion and flexibility, leaders and organizations that embrace cultural intelligence will be the ones that truly succeed.

CQ is not an innate talent—it is a skill that can be cultivated and strengthened through deliberate effort, much like building physical fitness. Leclerc, Kennedy, and Campis (2023) describe CQ as a "muscle" that grows through intentional practice and exposure to diverse perspectives. This metaphor emphasizes the dynamic and developmental nature of CQ, encouraging individuals to actively engage in opportunities that challenge their existing worldview and expand their cultural competence. By committing to this practice, leaders can not only enhance their own ability to communicate and collaborate effectively but also inspire their teams to embrace diversity as a source of strength and innovation.

The Foundations of Cultural Intelligence

Cultural intelligence (CQ) is a framework harnessing the power of the shared human experience. It's designed to help individuals and leaders navigate the complexities of cross-cultural interactions. It equips people to communicate effectively, foster collaboration, and build stronger relationships in diverse environments. At its core, CQ comprises four key components: CQ Drive, CQ Knowledge, CQ Strategy, and CQ Action. Each plays a unique role in enhancing cultural adaptability, yet it is their interconnectedness that drives meaningful communication and collaboration.

Cultural Intelligence Drive: Motivation to Engage with Cultural Diversity

CQ Drive represents the motivation and interest to interact with people from different cultural backgrounds. This component is rooted in curiosity and openness, encouraging individuals to embrace cultural diversity as an opportunity rather than a challenge. When people have a high CQ Drive, they exhibit a willingness to step outside their comfort zones, engage with unfamiliar cultures, and build genuine connections. For leaders, CQ Drive is essential for creating inclusive environments where diverse perspectives are valued. It sets the foundation for effective communication by fostering trust and respect, paving the way for fruitful interactions.

Cultural Intelligence Knowledge: Understanding Cultural Norms, Values, and Differences

CQ Knowledge refers to the understanding of how cultures differ in their norms, values, and communication styles. This component enables individuals to identify and appreciate the nuances that shape behavior across cultural contexts. For example, CQ Knowledge might involve recognizing the importance of hierarchy in one culture and the emphasis on egalitarianism in another. By grasping these cultural dimensions, individuals can avoid misunderstandings, adjust their expectations, and engage in conversations that resonate with the other party's values. Leaders with high CQ Knowledge are better equipped to tailor their communication approaches, ensuring their messages are meaningful and culturally appropriate.

Cultural Intelligence Strategy: Planning and Monitoring Cross-Cultural Interactions

CQ Strategy involves the ability to prepare for and reflect on cross-cultural interactions. This component encourages individuals to anticipate potential cultural differences, strategize how to navigate them, and evaluate the effectiveness of their communication afterward. CQ Strategy is particularly valuable in team settings, where diverse viewpoints can lead to both innovation and conflict (Andresen & Bergdolt, 2017). By employing this forward-thinking approach, leaders can proactively address challenges, foster collaboration, and ensure that interactions align with organizational goals. CQ Strategy transforms communication into a thoughtful and intentional process, enhancing its impact and reducing the likelihood of missteps.

Cultural Intelligence Action: Adapting Behavior to Different Cultural Contexts

CQ Action is the practical application of cultural intelligence—adapting one's behavior to suit the norms and expectations of different cultural contexts. This component involves flexibility and responsiveness, enabling individuals to adjust their communication styles, tone, and mannerisms based on cultural cues. Whether it's a leader adjusting their presentation style to align with a collectivist audience or a team member navigating varying approaches to decision-making, CQ Action ensures interactions remain respectful and effective. It is the execution phase where the other components—Drive, Knowledge, and Strategy—translate into tangible results, making communication dynamic and adaptable (Figure 8).

The Interconnection of Cultural Intelligence Components

The four components of CQ—Drive, Knowledge, Strategy, and Action—are deeply interconnected, reflecting the essential interplay of Being, Knowing, and Doing. CQ Drive embodies *Being*, the intrinsic motivation and openness to engage with cultural

FIGURE 8
The Four Components of Cultural Intelligence.
The four components of Cultural Intelligence align with the foundational framework of Being, Knowing, and Doing.

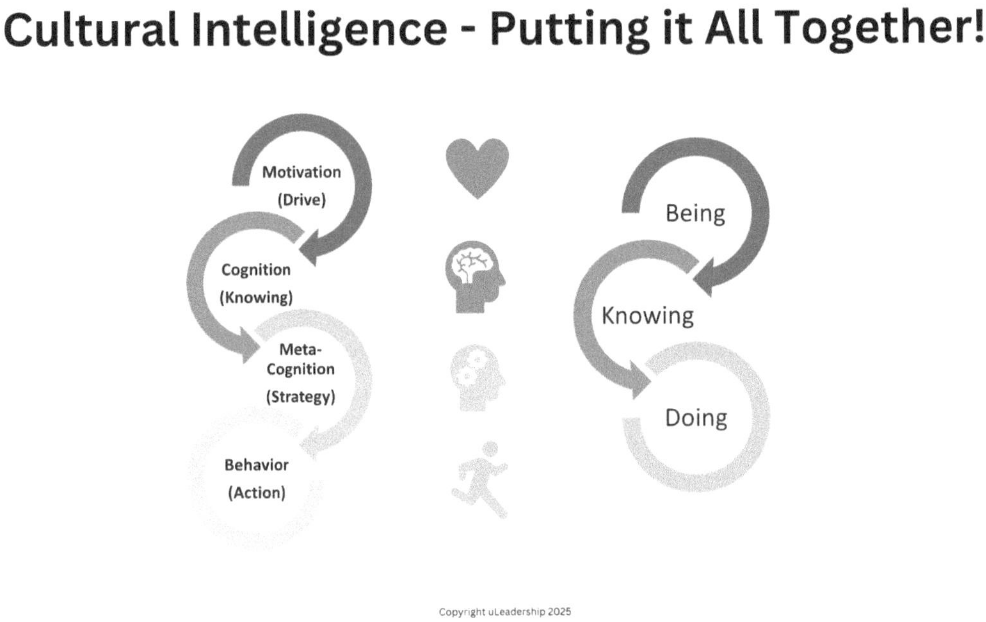

diversity, setting the foundation for genuine curiosity and respect. CQ Knowledge represents *Knowing*, the intellectual grasp of cultural norms, values, and differences that empowers individuals to approach interactions with informed sensitivity. CQ Strategy and CQ Action reflect *Doing*, as they translate knowledge and motivation into tangible behaviors—planning effectively and adapting with agility to cross-cultural contexts. Together, these components form a comprehensive framework that fosters respectful, meaningful, and impactful communication. By integrating Being, Knowing, and Doing, individuals and leaders can cultivate cultural intelligence as a dynamic force, enabling them to navigate diversity, inspire collaboration, and unlock innovation through deeper human connections.

Bridging Differences Through Communication

CQ enables leaders to navigate cultural differences with empathy, adaptability, and respect, ensuring that communication is effective and inclusive. By recognizing the common threads of humanity—universal emotions and shared experiences—nurse leaders can foster environments where diversity is celebrated as a strength rather than a barrier.

Empathy and active listening are key to overcoming cultural barriers, as they allow individuals to connect with others on a deeper level. Empathy involves understanding and valuing the perspectives, feelings, and experiences of others, while active listening ensures that voices are truly heard and respected. For nurse leaders managing multicultural teams, practicing empathy may involve acknowledging cultural norms and values that influence team dynamics, while active listening allows team members to share their unique viewpoints openly. This combination builds trust and psychological safety, creating a foundation for collaboration and innovation.

The universality of human emotions and shared experiences further reinforces CQ as a powerful tool for leaders. While cultural differences may shape how emotions are expressed, the essence of feelings such as joy, grief, and hope remains consistent across all cultures. Nurse leaders can leverage this universality to foster connections, using shared experiences to build common ground within diverse teams. For example, recognizing the collective challenges faced in patient care—such as addressing emotional distress or celebrating recovery milestones—can unify multicultural teams around their shared purpose and goals.

One practical healthcare example involves a nurse leader managing a team with members from various cultural backgrounds. By applying CQ, the leader could hold regular team meetings to encourage open dialogue, actively listen to each team member's perspective, and foster empathy by sharing stories of common challenges encountered in patient care. The leader could also use their cultural knowledge to address misunderstandings respectfully and adapt communication styles to match cultural preferences. This approach not only strengthens collaboration within the team but also enhances patient outcomes by ensuring culturally sensitive care practices.

Cultural intelligence provides nurse leaders with the ability to bridge differences and foster meaningful communication within multicultural teams. Through empathy, active listening, and recognizing shared human experiences, leaders can create inclusive environments where diversity becomes a powerful asset. CQ equips nurse leaders to adapt effectively, address challenges constructively, and ultimately inspire teams to excel in delivering compassionate, patient-centered care. It is not merely a skill to develop but a mindset to embrace, offering profound opportunities to enhance relationships and collective impact.

The Impact of Cultural Intelligence on Collaboration and Innovation

CQ plays a pivotal role in fostering collaboration and innovation within healthcare and nursing leadership. Recognizing and respecting cultural diversity enables teams to function more cohesively and generate creative solutions to complex problems. In healthcare settings, where professionals from different cultural backgrounds often work together, CQ equips nurse leaders to create an environment where every individual feels valued and heard. By embracing diverse perspectives, nurse leaders can encourage team members to share unique insights, resulting in more innovative approaches to patient care and operational challenges. Respecting cultural diversity also helps reduce misunderstandings and conflicts, enabling teams to focus on shared goals with greater efficiency.

One scenario that illustrates the impact of CQ involves a nurse leader managing a multicultural team in a large hospital. This leader recognized that communication styles varied significantly among team members due to cultural differences. By leveraging CQ, the leader implemented structured team meetings, ensuring active listening and inclusive discussions. Additionally, the leader conducted cultural awareness workshops to promote mutual understanding. As a result, the team collaboratively developed a patient care protocol tailored to the needs of a diverse patient population. This approach not only improved the team's cohesion and trust but also led to enhanced patient outcomes, as the protocol addressed cultural sensitivities that had previously been overlooked. Similar successes have been observed across other industries, where culturally intelligent leadership has driven research, expanded innovation, and strengthened collaboration (Ang, Van Dyne, & Rockstuhl, 2015).

The downstream effects of CQ extend beyond immediate teamwork and innovation, significantly impacting quality, safety, and job satisfaction in healthcare. Teams led by culturally intelligent nurse leaders often experience higher levels of psychological safety, where individuals feel empowered to speak up about potential risks or ideas for improvement (Remtulla et al., 2021). This open communication leads to better patient care practices and a reduction in errors. Moreover, fostering an inclusive and respectful workplace culture enhances job satisfaction and retention, as team members feel valued and supported. Ultimately, CQ not only strengthens collaboration and innovation but also creates a ripple effect that elevates the overall performance and well-being of both healthcare teams and the patients they serve.

Strengthening Your Cultural Intelligence Muscle

Developing CQ is a dynamic and intentional process that empowers individuals to adapt effectively to diverse cultural contexts. Strengthening the CQ "muscle" involves consistent practice, self-reflection, and engagement with experiences that challenge existing perspectives. For nurse leaders managing multicultural teams, enhancing CQ is particularly crucial for fostering inclusivity, collaboration, and innovation. Practical strategies such as self-assessment tools, reflective practices, and role-playing exercises provide a robust framework for growth, enabling leaders to navigate cultural differences with confidence and empathy.

Self-assessment tools, such as the CQ Self-Assessment referenced by Leclerc et al. (2023), are instrumental in building awareness of one's cultural intelligence strengths and areas for improvement. These tools evaluate key components such as CQ Drive, CQ Knowledge, CQ Strategy, and CQ Action, helping individuals pinpoint strengths and gaps in their cultural adaptability. For nurse leaders, starting with Self means utilizing self-assessment to gain insight into their leadership style and communication approaches within diverse teams. Now, it's your turn! As part of the Reflection for this chapter, we're challenging you to take the Human-Centered CQ Self-Assessment (Leclerc et al., 2023). These insights will serve you well as a foundation for targeted growth, offering a clear path to enhance your ability to engage meaningfully across the shared human continuum.

Reflective practices are equally vital in developing CQ, as they encourage us to examine our own biases and assumptions. Nurse leaders can engage in reflective practices by journaling, seeking feedback, or participating in discussions that highlight cultural differences and commonalities. When you take the Human-Centered CQ Self-Assessment, be sure to examine those areas where you may need to do some work. We're all a work-in-progress and being able to call out our own biases, assumptions, and potential blind spots will make us stronger human-centered communicators. Also, reflecting on past interactions allows us to identify moments where cultural misunderstandings may have occurred and strategize ways to improve communication. Over time, these practices cultivate a mindset of empathy and openness, empowering leaders to approach cross-cultural challenges with greater sensitivity and insight.

Role-playing and simulation exercises provide hands-on opportunities to practice cultural adaptability in real-world scenarios. These exercises immerse nurse leaders and teams in situations that mimic cross-cultural interactions, allowing them to

Human-Centered CQ Self-Assessment—Your Turn!

Rate the extent to which you agree with each statement, using the scale:

1 = strongly disagree, 2 = disagree, 3 = neutral, 4 = agree, 5 = strongly agree.

Motivational CQ

Lead with *Curiosity*! Explore how your level of interest, persistence, and confidence drive cultural interactions.

___ I am naturally curious and interested in learning about unfamiliar cultures of colleagues and patients.

___ I feel confident when interacting with patients and colleagues from a culture new to me.

___ I actively seek experiences in which I can immerse myself in interactions and dialogue with patients and colleagues who have different cultures.

___ I am persistent in interacting with patients and colleagues of different cultures even if I'm struggling to communicate.

___ I seek resources to facilitate successful and positive interactions with patients and colleagues of cultures new to me.

Total ___/5 = Motivational CQ

Cognitive CQ

Knowledge is power! Identify your level of understanding and awareness about how cultures are similar and different.

___ If I know I'm going to be interacting with patients or colleagues of different cultures, I do some research to find out at least the basics about the culture.

___ I take what I learn from cultural interactions with patients and colleagues and integrate it into how I'll approach people of other cultures in the future.

___ I put intentional thought into what I want to achieve from interactions with patients and colleagues of other cultures.

___ I mindfully pause before interacting with patients or colleagues of other cultures to check my own assumptions and biases.

___ If I encounter patients and colleagues of other cultures without time to prepare or pause, I lead with curiosity to learn cultural similarities and differences from the person or family.

Total _______/5 = Cognitive CQ

Behavioral CQ

Actions may speak as loud as your words! Reflect on your ability to adapt when relating and working with different cultures.

___ I easily adapt my body language to align with the expected norms of patients' and colleagues' cultures, e.g., eye contact, physical distance.

___ I easily modify my speech style to align with the expected norms of patients' and colleagues' cultures, e.g., tone, speed of speech.

___ I readily negotiate with patients or colleagues to honor cultural practices within the healthcare setting, e.g., prayer times, artifacts for cultural practices.

___ I practice mindfulness in my interactions with colleagues and patients bringing my full attention to the moment to honor their voice and see them as unique humans.

___ I am self-aware in harmonizing and honoring the cultural practices of patients and colleagues while doing the same for my own cultural practices.

Total ___/5 = Behavioral CQ

Note: Adapted from Early and Mosakowski (2004).

experiment with various communication styles and behaviors. For instance, a role-playing session might involve navigating a disagreement between team members with contrasting cultural norms. By actively engaging in such exercises, leaders can develop practical skills and adaptability, reinforcing their ability to respond effectively in diverse settings while building psychological safety within teams.

Ultimately, nurse leaders who model CQ behaviors set a powerful example for their teams, fostering a culture of inclusivity and respect. By actively demonstrating empathy, reflective thinking, and adaptability, leaders inspire their team members to embrace diversity as a strength. This leadership approach creates a ripple effect, encouraging collaboration, innovation, and trust within the workplace. Strengthening CQ is not only a personal journey but also a collective effort that transforms organizational culture and drives meaningful impact in multicultural healthcare environments.

TAKEAWAYS

- You're more likely to be effective at working and relating with others who are different from you if you *WANT* to be . . . spark your **motivation** to *DRIVE* your CQ!
- Harness your **cognition** superpower . . . think *DIFFERENTLY* about how we're the same and how we're different!
- Use **metacognition** to be *MINDFUL* and in the moment . . . make a plan and strategy to work your CQ muscle!
- Walk the talk! **Behaviors** illustrate *ACTION* and often, actions speak louder than words.

Final Thoughts

CQ is not just a theoretical concept; it is a vital skill that transforms human-centered communication into a powerful tool for building bridges across cultural divides. In healthcare and leadership, CQ enables individuals to foster trust, respect, and understanding in environments where diversity is the norm. By embracing the principles of empathy, active listening, and adaptability, nurse leaders and professionals alike can enhance teamwork, innovation, and patient outcomes. As this chapter has demonstrated, the components of CQ—Drive, Knowledge, Strategy, and Action—offer a practical framework for navigating the complexities of multicultural contexts with sensitivity and confidence.

The journey toward strengthening CQ begins with intentionality and commitment. Whether through self-assessment tools, reflective practices, or hands-on simulation exercises, taking the first step is key to developing this influential skill. Leaders have a unique opportunity to model CQ behaviors, creating inclusive environments where diversity is celebrated as a source of strength. By making cultural intelligence a priority, organizations can inspire meaningful collaboration, unlock creative solutions, and foster deeper human connections. It's time to flex your CQ muscle and lead the way in bridging cultural differences for a more inclusive and impactful future.

Discussion Questions for Groups

1. How do emotional intelligence and CQ complement each other in the context of healthcare leadership? Discuss how nurse leaders can leverage both emotional intelligence and CQ to build trust, resolve conflicts, and enhance team cohesion in multicultural healthcare environments.
2. What strategies can nurse leaders implement to cultivate CQ within their teams and ensure that culturally sensitive care practices are consistently integrated into patient care? Reflect on potential barriers and opportunities in fostering a culturally intelligent healthcare team.

Reflection Questions for Individuals

Take the Human-Centered CQ Self-Assessment to get an idea of your strengths and areas for growth.

1. What are your areas of strength?
2. What are your areas for growth?
3. Which component would you like to improve?
4. Reflect and commit to one strategy you can put in place to take a step toward improving your CQ.

References

Andresen, M., & Bergdolt, F. (2017). A systematic review on the definitions of global mindset and cultural intelligence—merging two different research streams. *The International Journal of Human Resource Management, 28*(1), 170–195. http://doi.org/10.1080/09585192.2016.1243568

Ang, S., Van Dyne, L., & Rockstuhl, T. (2015). Cultural intelligence: Origins, conceptualization, evolution, and methodological diversity. In M. J. Gelfand, C. Y. Chiu, & Y. Y. Hong (Eds.), *Handbook of advances in culture and psychology* (Vol. 5, pp. 273–323). Oxford University Press.

Early, P. C., & Mosakowski, E. (2004, October). Cultural intelligence. *Harvard Business Review, 82*(10), 139–146. Retrieved from https://hbr.org/2004/10/cultural-intelligence

Leclerc, L., Kennedy, K., & Campis, S. (2023). Cultural intelligence (CQ): Flex your CQ muscle through a Human-Centered Leadership workout! *Nurse Leader, 21*(3), 362–365.

Remtulla, R., Hagana, A., Houbby, N., Ruparell, K., Aojula, N., Menon, A., . . . Meyer, E. (2021). Exploring the barriers and facilitators of psychological safety in primary care teams: A qualitative study. *BMC Health Services Research, 21*, 269. doi: 10.1186/s12913-021-06232-7

Recommended Reading

Early, P. C., & Peterson, R. S. (2004). The elusive cultural chameleon: Cultural intelligence as a new approach to intercultural training for the global manager. *Academy of Management Learning and Education, 3*(1), 100–115.

Ott, D. L., & Michailova S. (2018). Cultural intelligence: A review and new research avenues. *International Journal of Management Reviews, 20*(1), 99–119. doi: 10.1111/ijmr.12118

Ramroop, M. (2021). *The inclusive culture pyramid. Implementing CQ as an EDI/DEI solution in organisations.* White Paper. Cultural Intelligence Center. Retrieved from https://culturalq.com/white-paper-the-inclusive-culture-pyramid/?source=case_studies

CHAPTER 12

Affirmative Disruption

Challenging the Status Quo

Influential people are never satisfied with the status quo. They're the ones who constantly ask, "What if?" and "Why not?" They're not afraid to challenge conventional wisdom and they don't disrupt things for the sake of being disruptive; they do it to make things better.

—Travis Bradberry, American author

Disruption often gets a bad rap—it sounds chaotic, unsettling, and even reckless. But affirmative disruption flips that idea on its head. Instead of tearing things down just for the sake of change, it's about challenging outdated norms with purpose and optimism. Healthcare, like many industries, is shaped by deeply ingrained traditions. Some of these structures provide stability, but others create barriers to growth, communication, and inclusivity. That's where Human-Centered Leadership (HCL) comes in—it prioritizes people, relationships, and transparency, making it the perfect foundation for affirmative disruption. When leaders embrace intentional, ethical disruption, they create space for innovation while keeping patients, teams, and communities at the heart of every decision.

One of the biggest hurdles to change? Inertia. Systems resist movement, and people can hesitate to step outside of familiar ways of thinking. But transformation doesn't have to feel like a battle—it can thrive on optimism, trust, and collaboration. In healthcare, where lives are literally on the line, leaders must disrupt strategically. Shaking up traditional communication norms—ditching hierarchy in favor of transparency—allows ideas to flow and voices to be heard. Likewise, fostering adaptability creates environments where meaningful change isn't just possible, but sustainable. At its core, affirmative disruption isn't just about shaking things up—it's about leading boldly toward a future where innovation and humanity go hand in hand.

The Foundation of Affirmative Disruption: Non-Zero-Sum Game (Self)

Affirmative disruption isn't about shaking things up just for the sake of change—it's about challenging outdated norms with purpose, inclusivity, and ethics (Fairbank, 2020). Healthcare, with its deeply ingrained traditions, often resists transformation, making it even more crucial that disruption be thoughtful and human-centered. At the heart of this approach lies Self, one of the key dimensions of HCL, which emphasizes self-awareness and mindfulness. Leaders who practice self-awareness understand their own biases, assumptions, and emotional triggers, allowing them to disrupt thoughtfully rather than reactively. Mindfulness ensures that change isn't rushed or reckless—it's intentional, responsive, and deeply connected to the realities of healthcare teams and patients. When disruption is grounded in self-awareness, it fosters environments where innovation and humanity thrive together, rather than causing unnecessary upheaval.

One of the biggest misconceptions about disruption is that it must be aggressive—forceful enough to break old systems apart. But in reality, the most effective change happens when leaders balance boldness with reflection. Disruption must be deliberate and ethical, meaning leaders must consistently ask: Which norms are holding us back? Which systems reinforce exclusion instead of inclusion? How can we disrupt in ways that empower rather than destabilize? When leaders cultivate mindfulness, they approach these questions with clarity and strategic foresight, ensuring that change strengthens patient care, builds trust, and supports team collaboration rather than fueling resistance.

A great example of affirmative disruption in action is the difference between zero-sum versus non-zero-sum thinking in healthcare. In a zero-sum approach, people believe that gains come at the expense of others—if resources are allocated to one team, another must suffer. This often leads to territorialism, competition, and resentment

Affirmative Disruption calls for a Non-Zero-Sum approach where a shared mindset of collaboration creates a win-win situation. Human-centered leaders are Non-Zero-Sum disrupters.

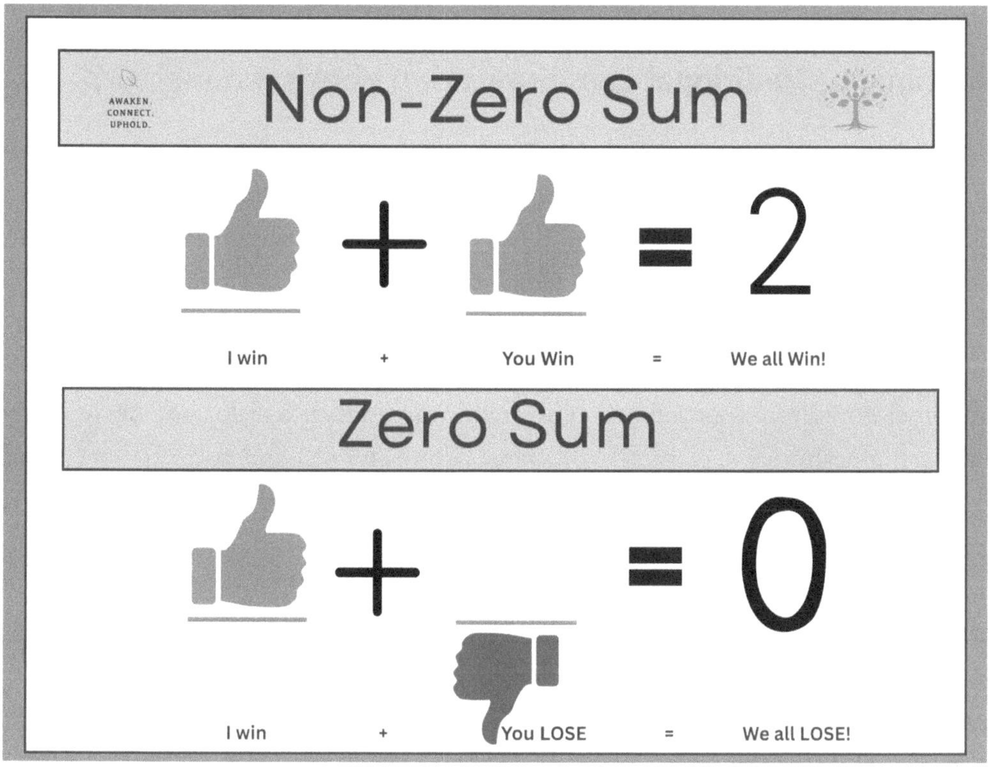

between departments, ultimately stifling collaboration and harming patient care. Now, contrast that with a non-zero-sum mindset, where leaders recognize that shared success leads to better outcomes for everyone. Imagine a hospital where the emergency department and the medical–surgical unit once operated in silos, each protecting their own processes. But through affirmative disruption—led by a self-aware, mindful leader—the teams shift toward collaborative decision-making, reducing inefficiencies and improving patient transitions in care. Instead of competing for influence, they realize that working together leads to better care, reduced burnout, and a stronger organizational culture.

Ultimately, affirmative disruption isn't about tearing down the old—it's about rebuilding with purpose. Leaders who embrace self-awareness and mindfulness create spaces where people feel safe to challenge norms, knowing their concerns will be heard rather than dismissed. When disruption is grounded in optimism and trust, it becomes unstoppable, shaping workplaces where creativity thrives, healthcare professionals feel valued, and systems evolve to truly serve the needs of diverse communities. By rejecting zero-sum thinking and fostering non-zero collaboration, leaders ensure that disruption moves healthcare toward a future that is inclusive, adaptive, and deeply human.

Rethinking Traditional Communication Norms (Connector)

For too long, communication in healthcare has followed a rigid, top-down structure—leaders dictate, frontline workers comply, and patients navigate a system that often feels impersonal. But Human-Centered Leadership in Healthcare (HCL-HC) challenges this model, emphasizing the Connector, where leaders actively build bridges between individuals, teams, and diverse perspectives. Effective communication isn't just about delivering information; it's about creating shared understanding. This means shifting from transactional conversations to authentic dialogues, where voices across the healthcare spectrum—clinicians, administrators, and patients—are heard and valued. The Connector mindset recognizes that great ideas come from every level of an organization, not just leadership. Remember, Connectors are like Michelangelo looking for the angel, or the David, in the marble! When leaders say, "I trust you," they empower teams to take ownership of communication, fostering an environment where clarity, engagement, and collaboration replace hierarchy and hesitation.

One of the biggest obstacles to meaningful communication is fear—the fear of speaking up, of challenging authority, or of navigating difficult conversations. But affirmative disruption thrives in environments where tough discussions aren't avoided; they're embraced as opportunities for growth (Fairbank, 2020). Crucial conversations—whether about patient safety, organizational change, or interpersonal conflicts—need to be handled with clarity, respect, and a willingness to listen. In HCL, Authentic Communication ensures these discussions go beyond surface-level exchanges. Leaders must set the tone for transparency, making it clear that disagreement isn't a threat but a catalyst for improvement. When done well, difficult conversations transform relationships, strengthening accountability and innovation instead of fueling resentment or resistance.

Conflict is inevitable in healthcare—high-stakes environments, diverse perspectives, and competing priorities naturally lead to tension. However, traditional approaches to conflict often focus on control rather than resolution. HCL-HC reframes conflict management, treating it as a constructive process rather than a disruption to workflow. Instead of avoiding disagreements, leaders act as Connectors, guiding teams toward mutual understanding and shared solutions. Whether mediating between departments, navigating ethical dilemmas, or resolving interpersonal clashes, effective leaders facilitate conversations that prioritize empathy and problem-solving over blame. This approach encourages teams to see conflict as a pathway to stronger collaboration, rather than something to be feared or suppressed.

A real-world example of this shift can be seen in a hospital's transition from hierarchical patient rounding structures to interdisciplinary rounds. In the traditional, hierarchical model, nurses felt hesitant to offer feedback about their patients, fearing their input wouldn't be valued. But a newly appointed chief medical officer—a strong Connector—recognized the untapped excellence in the nursing teams and worked with nursing, pharmacy, and therapy teams to implement interdisciplinary rounds, where frontline nurses, physicians, pharmacists, and therapists could voice concerns without fear. Over time, throughput improved, staff engagement increased, and communication became more fluid, respectful, and solution-driven. By trusting the expertise of all team members, this leader transformed communication from a one-way directive into a collaborative dialogue, proving that rethinking communication norms is a catalyst for innovation.

Ultimately, rethinking traditional communication norms isn't just about improving workflows—it's about creating cultures of trust, inclusion, and adaptability. Healthcare leaders who embrace authentic communication set the foundation for deeper engagement, ensuring conversations become tools for connection rather than barriers to progress. Affirmative disruption pushes past outdated norms, challenging hierarchies that stifle honest dialogue and replacing them with structures that encourage transparency. When leaders model openness, when teams feel safe to express concerns, and when communication is treated as a shared responsibility, healthcare environments evolve in ways that benefit both professionals and the patients they serve.

Challenging Inertia—Cultivating a Culture of Change (Upholder)

Change is hard—especially in healthcare, where routines and deeply ingrained traditions often dictate how things are done. Inertia can be comforting, giving organizations a sense of stability, but when it prevents innovation or stifles progress, it becomes a roadblock to growth. Inertia isn't just a healthcare issue. How many of you have heard of Kodak or Blockbuster? For the Gen Xers and Boomers in the audience, you'll vividly remember that Kodak was the source of film for printing our beloved pictures. While Kodak was busy spending money and time to protect its existing business, they failed to embrace the potential of digital technology (Anthony, 2016). We all know how that ended. We can't imagine a world without our phone at the ready with all of our pictures! Blockbuster followed the same path and died a slow digital death by betting against streaming services such as Netflix (Satell, 2014). Leaders who embrace affirmative disruption know that challenging inertia, like film and VHS tapes, isn't just about introducing new ideas like digital pictures and streaming; it's about cultivating a culture where change feels possible and safe. This is where psychological safety comes in—people need to feel secure enough to question norms, voice concerns, and experiment without fear of backlash. When leaders prioritize trust and openness, teams become more willing to engage in transformation rather than resist it.

The Upholder dimension of HCL-HC plays a crucial role in fostering this environment. Upholders don't see change as a top-down mandate; they recognize that transformation must be collectively built. They are socially and organizationally aware and attuned to the realities of their teams—especially when inertia is fueled by fear, burnout, or a lack of ownership over change. Instead of pushing change onto resistant individuals, Upholders meet people where they are, offering empathy, clarity, and shared accountability. Their mindset is inclusive—they don't impose a vision, but instead cultivate it through deep listening, asking questions, and ensuring that every team member feels seen, heard, and valued. Disrupting inertia isn't just about fixing inefficiencies; it's about building trust in the process.

One major barrier to challenging inertia is the assumption that "this is just how things are"—the belief that certain systems, workflows, or communication norms are immovable. However, leaders who cultivate a culture of adaptability break this cycle by encouraging teams to question assumptions and reimagine possibilities. Conflict is inevitable in this process, as different viewpoints emerge, but when approached with transparency and constructive dialogue, disagreements become opportunities rather than obstacles. The ability to navigate crucial conversations with authenticity and fairness allows leaders to push through resistance without alienating those who fear change.

One real-world example of an Upholder cultivating caring change comes from a pediatric intensive care unit struggling with high stress and emotional exhaustion among nurses. Traditionally, decision-making was hierarchical, leaving frontline workers feeling unheard and emotionally drained. The new chief nursing officer, acting as an Upholder, shifted the culture by embedding peer support networks and collaborative care rounds where nurses could openly discuss patient challenges, ethical dilemmas, and personal struggles without fear of judgment. She didn't just implement policies—she showed her team, *"I see you. I value what you bring."* Over time, the culture transformed from reactive to proactive, where speaking up for change wasn't just an individual expectation but a shared commitment. Nurses reported higher engagement, reduced burnout, and stronger emotional well-being, leading to better patient care and a more connected team dynamic. Think about this example as a way to move toward not just a culture of change, but a culture of *caring* change.

Ultimately, disrupting inertia isn't about dismantling everything at once—it's about creating momentum in a way that feels sustainable and inclusive. Leaders who challenge the status quo with optimism, awareness, and psychological safety empower their teams to step forward with confidence. When people believe their contributions matter and when they feel encouraged to experiment, innovate, and rethink outdated norms, healthcare shifts from being stuck in tradition to thriving in evolution. Change isn't the enemy—it's the key to better patient care, stronger collaboration, and a system that reflects the real needs of the communities it serves.

Optimism as a Catalyst for Transformation (Awakener)

Optimism isn't just about seeing the bright side—it's about believing in possibility, even when faced with obstacles. In healthcare, where burnout, bureaucracy, and resistance to change can weigh down even the most motivated leaders, optimism serves as a powerful catalyst for transformation (Beute & Pacinelli, 2021). Leaders who embrace affirmative disruption recognize that change starts with mindset—the ability to look beyond limitations and see potential in individuals, teams, and the system itself. This is where the Awakener dimension of HCL-HC comes in. Awakeners inspire people to reimagine what's possible, offering coaching and mentorship that shifts perspectives from fear to opportunity. When leaders actively seek excellence in those around them, they fuel confidence, creativity, and a collective drive to build something better.

One of the most profound leadership tools? Four simple words: "I believe in you." It's incredible how much impact genuine encouragement can have on teams navigating uncertainty. Healthcare professionals often work under immense pressure, balancing patient care with systemic challenges. Without affirmation and support, doubt creeps in, innovation slows, and people settle into a routine rather than reaching for excellence. Leaders who mentor and coach with an optimistic mindset break this cycle—they create environments where people feel valued and empowered to bring forth new ideas, challenge outdated processes, and explore solutions that enhance patient care. By showing belief in their teams, leaders unlock a mindset shift, where challenges become opportunities rather than roadblocks.

Optimism also drives resilience, which is critical for navigating disruption. Healthcare systems don't change overnight, and resistance to new approaches is inevitable. Leaders who coach through transformation rather than dictate it strengthen the adaptability of their teams. Instead of dwelling on setbacks, optimistic leaders frame obstacles as learning moments, helping individuals refine their approach and remain committed to growth. Affirmative disruption isn't about forcing change—it's about cultivating trust, fostering belief in possibilities, and equipping people with the confidence to take bold steps forward.

One powerful example of a leader acting as an Awakener in healthcare comes from the transformation of a struggling emergency department. The department was plagued by inefficiencies, staff burnout, and poor patient satisfaction scores. Morale was low, and the team had adopted a zero-sum mindset, believing that improving patient flow meant sacrificing the well-being of clinicians. The department's human-centered nursing director, however, saw potential where others saw dead ends. Instead of imposing rigid top-down solutions, he coached and mentored his team to reimagine their workflow collaboratively.

He started by shifting the narrative, emphasizing a non-zero-sum approach—one where better patient care and improved working conditions could coexist. Through regular coaching sessions and genuine encouragement, he helped the staff see their own excellence and challenged them to come up with solutions. By fostering psychological safety, he made space for new ideas, including a team-based triage system that streamlined care without increasing stress. The result? Higher patient satisfaction, reduced wait times, and an energized, engaged team that felt ownership over the improvements they created.

In the end, optimism isn't just a feel-good sentiment—it's a strategy for lasting transformation. When healthcare leaders champion possibility over limitation, they create organizations where people thrive, creativity flourishes, and innovation accelerates. Awakener leaders set the tone by coaching, mentoring, and inspiring teams to see beyond the status quo. They look for excellence in individuals and teams and nurture it, ensuring that disruption isn't chaotic—it's visionary, intentional, and deeply human-centered. Transformation doesn't happen in isolation—it happens when leaders believe in their teams, their teams believe in themselves, and together, they believe in a better future.

Final Thoughts

Affirmative disruption isn't just about challenging the status quo—it's about leading with purpose, optimism, and inclusivity. The most effective leaders don't disrupt for the sake of change; they do it intentionally by fostering psychological safety, meaning-

TAKEAWAYS!

1. **Disrupt with purpose!** Bold leadership isn't about breaking things—it's about reimagining them with intention and optimism.
2. **Trust fuels transformation!** When leaders say, *"I believe in you. I trust you. I see you,"* teams feel empowered to challenge inertia and innovate.
3. **Communication is the game-changer!** Ditch hierarchy—transparent, authentic dialogue fosters collaboration and drives lasting change.
4. **Optimism is contagious!** Leaders who awaken excellence in others spark momentum, resilience, and a culture of forward-thinking innovation.
5. **Culture drives change!** Affirmative disruption isn't just about strategy—it's about creating workplaces where people feel valued, safe, and ready to lead transformation.

ful conversations, and trust within their teams. Here are some ways to challenge the status quo:

- Start by actively questioning outdated norms, ensuring that transformation empowers rather than destabilizes.
- Embrace transparent communication, encourage crucial conversations, and create space for innovation without fear.
- Most importantly, model HCL—whether as a Connector, Upholder, or Awakener—by recognizing excellence, valuing diverse perspectives, and championing authentic communication and trust.

Looking ahead, healthcare's future will be shaped by bold, optimistic leaders who refuse to settle for inertia. The industry doesn't just need technical advancements—it needs cultural transformation, where change is driven by empathy, adaptability, and human connection. Leaders who embrace affirmative disruption will cultivate cultures of trust, collaboration, and innovation, ensuring that patient care evolves alongside leadership practices. And at the heart of this evolution is HCL, a framework that ensures disruption isn't just about shaking up systems—it's about building environments where people feel valued, teams thrive, and the work itself is deeply meaningful.

In the end, affirmative disruption is a mindset, not just a strategy. It's the belief that healthcare can be more inclusive, more dynamic, and more innovative—and that transformation starts with leaders who see potential, trust their teams, and refuse to accept mediocrity. The challenge isn't just breaking old habits—it's leading a movement toward better care, stronger communities, and a future where healthcare is shaped by human connection and visionary leadership.

Discussion Questions for Groups

1. How can leaders ensure that affirmative disruption is both ethical and inclusive, rather than destabilizing? Consider real-world healthcare examples where disruption led to meaningful, positive change. What strategies helped create psychological safety and transparency during the process?
2. Optimism is framed as a catalyst for transformation in this chapter. How can healthcare leaders balance optimism with realism when challenging ingrained norms? Discuss situations where optimism was critical for overcoming inertia. How do trust-building (Connector) and mentorship (Awakener) influence how teams embrace disruption?

Reflection Questions for Individuals

1. How has inertia shaped your own leadership approach or workplace culture? Reflect on moments when you hesitated to challenge the status quo. What would it take to shift from resistance to affirmative disruption in a way that fosters trust and collaboration?

   ____

   ____

   ____

   ____

   ____

2. Think about a time when optimism influenced a difficult transition in healthcare or leadership. How did an optimistic leader (or your own mindset)

shape the outcome? How can you cultivate a balance between optimism and strategic realism to inspire meaningful change?

____

____

____

____

____

____

References

Anthony, S. D. (2016, July 15). Kodak's downfall wasn't about technology. *Harvard Business Review, 94*(7). Retrieved from https://hbr.org/2016/07/kodaks-downfall-wasnt-about-technology

Beute, E., & Pacinelli, S. (2021). *Human-centered communication.* Fast Company Press.

Fairbank, C. (2020, January 31). The importance of positive disruption in the workforce. Forbes. Retrieved from https://www.forbes.com/councils/forbescoachescouncil/2020/01/31/the-importance-of-positive-disruption-in-the-workforce

Satell, G. (2014, September 5). *A look back at why Blockbuster really failed and why it didn't have to.* Forbes. Retrieved from https://www.forbes.com/sites/gregsatell/2014/09/05/a-look-back-at-why-blockbuster-really-failed-and-why-it-didnt-have-to

Recommended Reading

Falikowski, A. (2002). *Mastering human relations* (4th ed., pp. 418–422). Pearson Education Canada.

Patterson, K., Grenny, J., McMillan, R., & Switzler, A. (2012). *Crucial conversations: Tools for talking when the stakes are high.* McGraw-Hill.

Rogers, E. M. (2003) *Diffusion of innovations* (5th ed.). Free Press.

Shaw, B., & Chisholm, O. (2020). Creeping through the backdoor: Disruption in medicine and health. *Frontiers in Pharmacology, 11*, 818.

Sounderajah, V., Patel, V., Varatharajan, L., Harling, L., Normahani, P., Symons, J., Barlow, J., Darzi, A., & Ashrafian, H. (2021). Are disruptive innovations recognised in the healthcare literature? A systematic review. *BMJ Innovations, 7*(1), 208–216.

Human-Centered Design

Human-Centered Design provides a framework for addressing complexity, fostering inclusivity, and prioritizing well-being in healthcare environments. *Systems thinking* helps leaders embrace interconnected challenges, ensuring solutions target root causes rather than symptoms. The *architecture of inclusion* transforms spaces and cultures by advancing equity and accessibility, ensuring all individuals feel valued. *Well-being by design* focuses on creating practice environments that nurture both patients and healthcare teams, reinforcing a supportive and sustainable workplace. Together with HCL-HC, these principles shape a healthcare system that is responsive, equitable, and designed with people at its core.

CHAPTER 13

Using Systems Thinking to Build Human-Centered Solutions

Business and human endeavors are systems . . . we tend to focus on snapshots of isolated parts of the system and wonder why our deepest problems never get solved.

—Peter Senge, Author of the Fifth Discipline

Healthcare is messy. Not in the sense of disorganization, but in its sheer complexity—countless moving parts, shifting priorities, and human lives at the center of every decision. That's why systems thinking is a game-changer. It's not about fixing problems one by one—it's about seeing the bigger picture, understanding how everything connects, and identifying root causes rather than just treating symptoms. When leaders embrace this mindset, they stop chasing quick fixes and start designing real, lasting solutions that transform patient care, team dynamics, and healthcare systems as a whole.

This is where Human-Centered Leadership (HCL) and Human-Centered Design (HCD) step in. Leaders who Awaken, Connect, and Uphold don't just manage systems—they shape them by fostering trust, inclusion, excellence, and collaboration (Leclerc, Kennedy, & Campis, 2021). And HCD ensures solutions aren't just theoretical; they're tested, refined, and built around the actual needs of real people (Melles, Albayrak, & Goossens, 2021). Together, these two frameworks give leaders the ability to navigate healthcare's complexity with empathy, strategic thinking, and creativity, ensuring that change is not just efficient, but human-centered.

Too often, healthcare falls into the trap of symptom-focused solutions—patching up problems instead of tackling the deeper systemic issues causing them. Systems thinking pushes us to step back, question assumptions, and look at the unseen forces shaping our decisions. When leaders approach challenges with optimism, adaptability, and an interdisciplinary mindset, they stop reacting and start innovating—building cultures where teams feel empowered to rethink how healthcare works (Landeiro et al., 2025). Because in the end, the best healthcare systems aren't just effective; they are responsive, resilient, and built on a foundation of trust and human connection.

Systems Thinking in Healthcare: Seeing the Bigger Picture

Preflection: Setting the Stage

Before diving into systems thinking, take a moment to reflect:

- **What do you think of when you hear the word "systems?"** Do you picture a network of interconnected parts working toward a common goal?
- **How are you situated in the healthcare system?** Consider your role—whether as a clinician, administrator, or patient—and how you interact with different components of care delivery.

These questions will help frame the discussion, encouraging you to see healthcare not as a collection of isolated tasks but as a complex, adaptive system where every decision, process, and relationship is interconnected.

What Is Systems Thinking?

Systems thinking is more than just a problem-solving tool—it's a mindset that helps leaders and teams see the whole picture rather than focusing on individual parts in isolation. Peter Senge, author of The Fifth Discipline (2006), describes it as a framework for seeing interrelationships rather than things, for seeing patterns of change rather than static snapshots. Similarly, Kim (1999) defines a system as a group of interacting, interrelated, or interdependent parts that form a unified whole with a specific purpose.

In healthcare, this means shifting from linear thinking—where problems are analyzed in isolation—to circular thinking, which recognizes feedback loops, adaptability, and interconnectedness. Instead of treating symptoms, systems thinking encourages leaders to identify root causes, ensuring that solutions address the deeper structures influencing outcomes.

Addressing Root Causes Versus Treating the Symptoms

Healthcare challenges often appear as isolated events—a sudden spike in patient readmissions, staff burnout, or inefficiencies in care delivery. But these events are just the tip of the iceberg. Beneath them lie patterns, underlying structures, and mental models that shape behaviors and outcomes.

- **Events**: The visible problems we react to (e.g., a medication error).
- **Patterns**: Recurring trends that indicate deeper systemic issues (e.g., frequent errors in a specific unit).
- **Underlying Structures**: The systems, workflows, and policies that contribute to these patterns (e.g., lack of standardized communication protocols).
- **Mental Models**: The beliefs and assumptions that influence decision-making (e.g., "We've always done it this way").

By applying HCL, leaders can awaken awareness of these deeper layers, connect teams to shared solutions, and uphold ethical, adaptive problem-solving approaches. Similarly, HCD ensures that solutions are co-created with stakeholders, addressing not just symptoms but the root causes of systemic challenges (Figure 9).

Bridging Leadership, Design, and Systems Thinking

Healthcare isn't just about processes and policies—it's about people. That's why systems thinking, when combined with HCL and HCD, has the power to create lasting, meaningful change. A healthcare system isn't just a collection of departments working in isolation—it's a complex adaptive system where interactions, feedback loops, and relationships shape outcomes. Traditional siloed thinking tends to keep solutions

FIGURE 9
The Iceberg Model helps us consider the visible and invisible influences on what often appear to be "isolated" events on the surface. As we dive deeper, we discover there's so much more below the surface that influences the events we see. Human-centered leaders navigate the complex healthcare system and the "above the waterline" issues by *awakening* awareness of the deeper layers, *connecting* teams to shared solutions, and *upholding* ethical, adaptive problem-solving approaches.

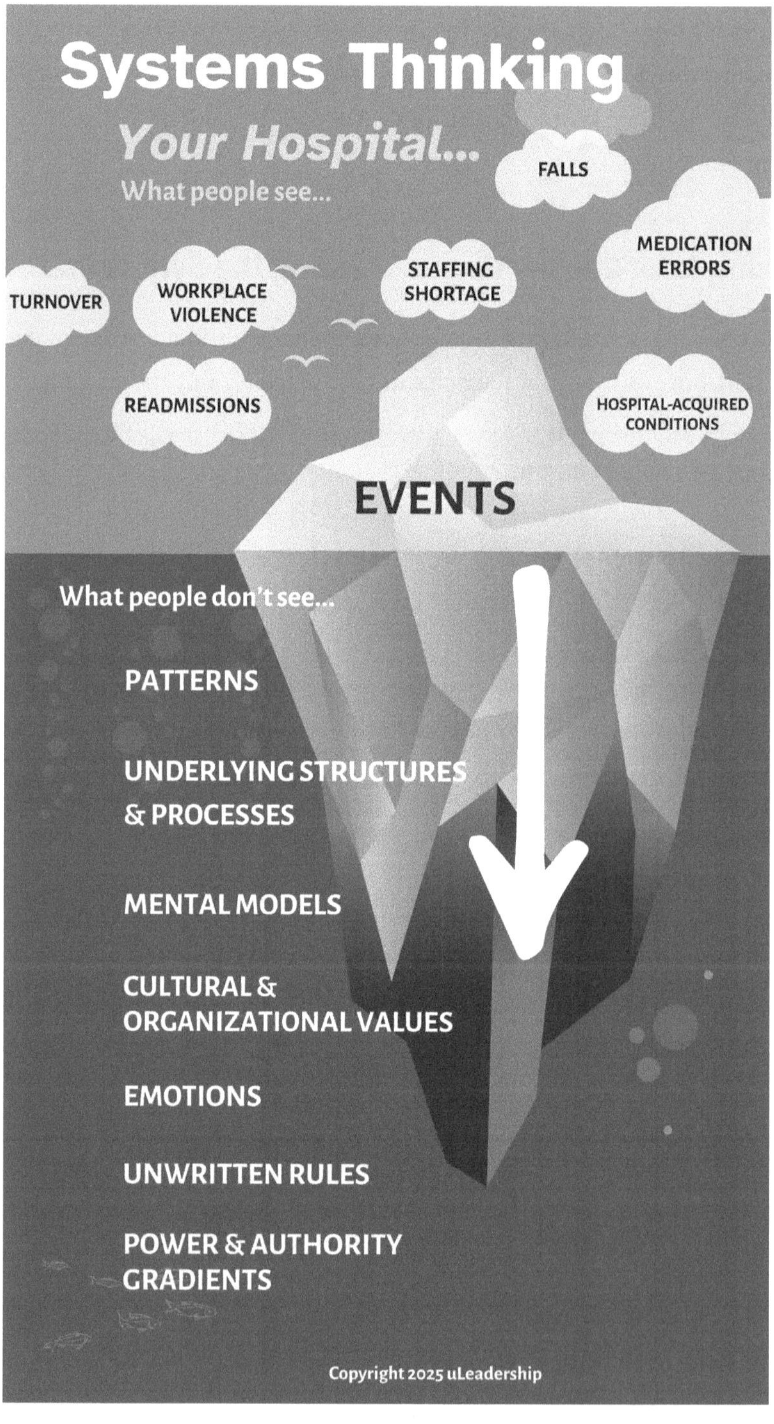

narrowly focused, addressing problems in isolation but leaders who embrace human-centered approaches recognize that collaboration, trust, and adaptability drive sustainable solutions. Instead of fixing single issues, they ask, "How do we rethink the system so it works better for the people in it?"

When healthcare leaders prioritize Awakening, Connecting, and Upholding, they see how individual choices, organizational design, and systemic forces intertwine. The best solutions don't come from rigid top-down decisions; they come from co-designing with the people directly impacted—patients, nurses, and frontline staff. That's where HCD steps in, giving teams the tools to prototype, refine, and implement solutions that respond to real-world needs. Whether it's addressing workplace violence or improving patient experience, leaders who listen first and design with empathy create systems that don't just function but thrive.

At its core, systems thinking in healthcare is all about connection. Decisions aren't just isolated choices—they ripple across departments, influence workflows, and shape patient care. Leaders who embrace feedback loops ensure that change isn't just theoretical—it's rooted in real human experiences. When healthcare shifts from reactive fixes to proactive, human-centered transformation, teams feel valued, empowered, and ready to shape a future that serves both individuals and the larger system. Because in the end, the best healthcare systems aren't just efficient—they're built on trust, inclusion, and a shared commitment to progress.

By integrating systems thinking, leaders move beyond quick fixes and create sustainable, meaningful change—ensuring that healthcare evolves to meet the needs of both individuals and the broader system. Look at the case example to see how it all comes together.

Leadership Habits for Systems Thinking in Healthcare

So how do we put action behind these great ideas for systems thinking and human-centered approaches? In a nutshell, we need to recognize that constantly putting out fires is just treating the symptoms. We need to pause long enough to see who or what is causing the fires in the first place. Effective leadership in healthcare isn't just about making quick decisions—it's about seeing the system as a whole while understanding how each moving part influences the bigger picture. Systems thinking leaders recognize that healthcare is deeply interconnected, meaning small adjustments can have widespread effects. They don't just focus on isolated events; instead, they look for patterns, trends, and underlying structures that shape long-term outcomes. The best leaders

CASE EXAMPLE

Using Systems Thinking and Human-Centered Approaches to Address Workplace Violence in Healthcare

The Challenge: A Surge in Workplace Violence

At a large urban hospital, incidents of workplace violence against nurses and staff had been steadily increasing. Reports showed physical assaults, verbal abuse, and threats from patients and visitors, leading to high turnover, burnout, and decreased morale among healthcare workers. Leadership initially responded with security measures, such as increased surveillance and stricter visitor policies, but the violence persisted.

Applying Systems Thinking

The hospital's chief nursing officer (CNO), recognizing that surface-level solutions weren't enough, decided to apply systems thinking using the *Iceberg Model* to uncover the *root causes* of the issue.

1. **Events (What is seen)**
   - Nurses reported frequent aggression from patients, especially in the emergency department.
   - Security interventions were reactive, addressing incidents after they occurred rather than preventing them.
2. **Patterns (Recurring trends)**
   - Violence was more common during peak hours when staff were overwhelmed.
   - Patients with mental health crises or substance use disorders were disproportionately involved in incidents.
   - Staff felt unsupported, fearing retaliation if they reported violence.
3. **Underlying Structures (Systemic causes)**
   - Lack of de-escalation training for frontline staff.
   - Inadequate mental health resources for patients in crisis.
   - Poor communication between departments leads to inconsistent responses to violent incidents.

CASE EXAMPLE

4. **Mental Models (Deep-seated beliefs)**
   - Some staff believed violence was "part of the job" and unavoidable.
   - Leadership had historically focused on punitive measures rather than preventative strategies.
   - Patients in distress were often seen as aggressors rather than individuals needing specialized care.

The Solution: A Human-Centered Approach

Using insights from Systems Thinking and Human-Centered Leadership in Healthcare, the CNO shifted the hospital's approach from reactive security measures to proactive, human-centered interventions:

- **Implemented de-escalation training** for all frontline staff, equipping them with techniques to manage aggression before it escalated.
- **Established a behavioral response team** to support staff in handling violent incidents with **trauma-informed care**.
- **Expanded mental health services**, including crisis intervention specialists in the emergency department.
- **Created a culture of psychological safety**, encouraging staff to report violence without fear of retaliation.
- **Redefined workplace violence policies**, ensuring clear protocols for prevention, intervention, and postincident support.

The Impact: A Safer, More Supportive Workplace

Within a year, the hospital saw a 40% reduction in violent incidents, improved staff morale, and higher retention rates. Nurses reported feeling more confident and supported, and patients in crisis received better care without escalating into violence. By addressing the deeper systemic issues, the CNO transformed workplace safety—not just through rules, but by changing mindsets, structures, and culture.

This case illustrates how systems thinking and human-centered approaches can uncover hidden causes of workplace violence, leading to sustainable, human-centered solutions.

also embrace adaptability—rather than sticking rigidly to old models, they're open to new perspectives and willing to challenge assumptions that might be holding their teams back.

To integrate systems thinking into daily leadership practices, leaders must commit to ongoing reflection and learning. Routine exercises such as stakeholder mapping help identify who is impacted by key decisions, ensuring that change doesn't happen in a vacuum. Data and feedback loops play a crucial role—leaders who actively seek input from diverse teams ensure that their strategies remain responsive to real-world challenges. And just as healthcare is continuously evolving, systems thinking leaders recognize the importance of course correction, adjusting their approaches as new insights emerge.

A great example of systems thinking in action comes from a hospital struggling with patient flow inefficiencies, you know, the dreaded length of stay issue. The leadership team initially tried isolated fixes, such as adjusting nurse scheduling or improving intake protocols, but these changes had limited impact. By taking a systems thinking approach, they zoomed out to examine the broader structures influencing delays, including interdepartmental communication breakdowns and mismatched incentives across units. Through collaborative problem-solving and interdisciplinary teamwork, they implemented a coordinated patient-centered care model—reducing bottlenecks, improving care quality, and strengthening engagement across departments.

The most effective systems thinking leaders shift from zero-sum to non-zero-sum mindsets, ensuring that change isn't about winners and losers but shared progress. They empower teams by facilitating the "power within," helping individuals recognize their own capabilities. They encourage "power with others," building coalitions and fostering collaboration to drive transformation. And rather than being controlled by external forces, they cultivate "power under control," ensuring that leadership decisions are intentional, ethical, and forward-thinking. These habits aren't just good leadership—they're essential for a healthcare system that thrives on connection, adaptability, and continuous improvement.

Habits of a Systems Thinking Leader

- **Sees the big picture** while understanding details.
- **Recognizes patterns, trends, and underlying structures** to uncover root causes.
- **Is open to changing perspectives** and challenging long-held assumptions.
- **Uses stakeholder mapping** to assess impact across the system.
- **Values data and feedback loops** to refine decision-making.

- **Embraces course correction** to continuously improve strategies.
- **Facilitates collaboration** to shift from reactive fixes to proactive solutions.

Final Thoughts

The future of healthcare leadership demands more than quick fixes—it calls for systems thinking, HCL, and intentional design to create lasting impact. Leaders must move beyond symptom-based solutions, looking deeper to uncover root causes and designing holistic, wide-reaching improvements that strengthen both patient care and organizational resilience. By shifting their perspective to see interconnections, feedback loops, and adaptive structures, healthcare leaders can build environments where teams thrive, innovation flourishes, and challenges are tackled at their core rather than just treated on the surface. Awakening to complexity, Connecting through trust and collaboration, and Upholding a shared vision ensure that healthcare systems don't just evolve—they transform with purpose.

Looking ahead, bold, optimistic leadership, fueled by HCD, will shape the next era of healthcare. The most effective leaders embrace complexity, seeing challenges not as obstacles but as opportunities for creative solutions. By fostering interdisciplinary collaboration, embedding psychological safety, and co-designing solutions that reflect real human needs, healthcare can become more adaptive, inclusive, and responsive to the communities it serves. This is a call to action: step forward, rethink assumptions, and lead with the mindset that innovation and humanity are inseparable. Awaken. Connect. Uphold. Because when leaders move beyond traditional boundaries, healthcare becomes not just a system—but a movement toward meaningful change.

Discussion Questions for Groups

1. How can systems thinking help healthcare leaders move beyond reactive problem-solving to create sustainable, human-centered improvements? Discuss examples where symptom-based fixes led to short-term relief but failed to address deeper systemic challenges. What strategies can leaders use to uncover root causes and design long-lasting solutions?
2. In what ways does HCL-HC foster interdisciplinary collaboration within complex healthcare systems? How can leaders balance individual expertise with collective decision-making to drive innovation? Share experiences where cross-functional teamwork led to better patient outcomes or improved workplace culture.

Reflection Questions for Individuals

1. Think about a challenge in your healthcare environment that seems to repeat itself. How might systems thinking help uncover the underlying structures and mental models contributing to the issue? What steps could you take to shift from symptom-based fixes to a more holistic, long-term solution?

   ____

   ____

   ____

   ____

   ____

2. Consider your leadership approach—how do you currently engage with complexity and change? In what ways could integrating HCD and leadership principles enhance collaboration, adaptability, and innovation in your work?

   ____

   ____

   ____

   ____

   ____

References

Kim, D. H. (1999) Introduction to system thinking. In *System thinking tools and applications.* Pegasus Communications, Inc.

Landeiro, F., Silva, M., Veiga e Moura, C., Martins, C., Miller, P., Ferraz, S., de Azevedo, A. P., Gancho, S., Rocha, L., Patrício, R., & Nunes, I. (2025). Human-centered design and maternity care: Is this a possible interplay? A systematic review. *BMC Pregnancy and Childbirth, 25*, Article 261.

Leclerc, L., Kennedy, K., & Campis, S. (2021). Human-centered leadership in health care: A contemporary nursing leadership theory generated via constructivist grounded theory. *Journal of Nursing Management, 29*(3), 294–310.

Melles, M., Albayrak, A., & Goossens, R. (2021). Innovating health care: Key characteristics of human-centered design. *International Journal for Quality in Health Care, 33*(Supplement1), 37–44.

Senge, P. M. (2006). *The fifth discipline: The art & practice of the learning organization.* Doubleday Business.

Recommended Reading

George, A. S., McConville, F. E., de Vries, S., Nigenda, G., Sarfraz, S., & McIsaac, M. (2020). Violence against female health workers is the tip of iceberg of gender power imbalances, *BMJ, 371*, m3546. doi: 10.1136/bmj.m3546

John, K., Flynn, D., & Armstrong, M. (2018) Co-designing behaviour change in healthcare. In C. Storni, K. Leahy, M. McMahon, P. Lloyd, & E. Bohemia (Eds.), *Design as a catalyst for change—DRS International Conference 2018, 25–28 June, Limerick, Ireland.* doi: 10.21606/drs.2018.317

Lahey, T. (2020). The bottom of the healthcare rationing iceberg. *New England Journal of Medicine, 283*, 2200–2201. doi: 10.1056/NEJMp2021953

Leitao, S., Manning, E., Greene, R. A., & Corcoran, P. (2022). On behalf of the Maternal Morbidity Advisory Group. Maternal morbidity and mortality: An iceberg phenomenon. *BJOG, 129*, 402–411.

CHAPTER 14

The Architecture of Inclusion

How Human-Centered Design Shapes Healthcare Spaces and Cultures

A deep sense of love and belonging is an irreducible need of all people. We are biologically, cognitively, physically, and spiritually wired to love, to be loved, and to belong. When those needs are not met, we don't function as we were meant to. We break. We fall apart. We numb. We ache. We hurt each other. We get sick.

—Brené Brown

In healthcare, fostering environments of inclusivity and belonging isn't just about policies or checkboxes—it's about intentional design and leadership that truly prioritize the human experience at every level. Human-Centered Design (HCD) ensures that the spaces we work in, the systems we build, and the workflows we navigate genuinely reflect the real needs of patients, families, healthcare professionals, and the communities we serve. It transforms inclusion from an aspirational goal into a lived, tangible reality.

Pair this with Human-Centered Leadership in Healthcare—a leadership approach that champions psychological safety, relational trust, and a shared sense of purpose—and we create workplaces where voices are amplified, connections are celebrated, and the deeply shared humanity of healthcare is honored. When healthcare professionals feel genuinely valued, supported, and seen, they are empowered to provide compassionate care that meets patients where they are.

Inclusion isn't just about opening the door—it's about ensuring that everyone truly belongs once inside, that their voices are heard, their contributions are recognized, and their presence is respected in every encounter.

The Power of Invitation

Have you ever received a calendar invitation to a meeting with an agenda filled with discussions about staffing, patient care workflows, and hospital policy? As a healthcare leader, you understand the weight of these decisions—not just for your team, but for the patients who rely on your expertise. Healthcare leadership transcends policies and procedures; it's about recognizing the people behind those decisions and ensuring they feel valued and empowered.

The day of the meeting arrives. You step into the room, find a seat at the table, and prepare to engage. On paper, you are included. You're present, part of the discussion, and granted the opportunity to listen. Yet, as the meeting unfolds, something unsettling begins to take shape. Conversations are happening, decisions are being made, but your expertise isn't acknowledged. You voice concerns—or try to—about nurse fatigue, patient safety, or workflow inefficiencies, but your words seem to evaporate into the air, unnoticed. The conversation moves forward as if you hadn't spoken at all.

When the meeting ends, you walk away feeling invisible, questioning whether your presence truly mattered. I've been in those meetings—present but not truly belonging. At times, I internalized the disconnect, wondering if I had somehow failed, or perhaps because I am not naturally vocal or assertive, my contributions were not seen as valuable. But as I grew in my leadership journey, I came to realize an essential truth: Belonging doesn't happen by chance. It must be cultivated with intention, because only through deliberate effort can we create spaces where every individual feels valued—and the foundation of belonging is inclusivity.

True inclusion goes beyond extending an invite—it requires a deliberate effort to cultivate an environment where every individual feels seen, heard, and valued before they even step into the room. A truly inclusive space ensures that every personality type has a voice, not just the most outspoken. It honors listening as much as speaking, recognizing that meaningful contributions come in many forms. Inclusion, at its core, must be intentional. Without purposeful inclusivity, belonging remains out of reach. When individuals are present but not empowered—when their voices are acknowledged yet carry no weight—then inclusion becomes nothing more than an empty gesture.

Just as a hospital thrives when its patients feel cared for, a healthcare team excels when its members feel they belong. The ability to foster belonging among providers has a ripple effect, improving collaboration, morale, and, ultimately, patient care. The difference between being invited and truly belonging is leadership's commitment to fostering psychologically safe spaces where individuals don't just attend meetings—they help shape them.

Inclusion Versus Belonging: Bridging the Gap

So, what is the difference between inclusion and belonging, and how does it help us support the basic human need of mattering? Leadership in healthcare often emphasizes inclusion, but inclusion alone is not the goal. If our peers and colleagues don't feel engaged, valued, and empowered, their presence at the table is symbolic, and not impactful.

Consider the key differences between these concepts. Inclusivity is the bedrock of belonging because it ensures that every individual is invited, whether it be to that important meeting or to be a part of the team. Inclusion is an action. However, leadership that stops at inclusion misses the opportunity to build truly effective and engaged teams. Belonging, on the other hand, is a feeling. When people feel like they belong to something, they feel safe to be and express their authentic selves.

Research suggests that recognizing and valuing others—even through simple gestures like using their names—can enhance self-esteem, cognitive function, and memory while reducing loneliness and burnout (Riddle & Métraux, 2021). Another study emphasized the need for psychologically safe cultures, where individuals feel seen, heard, and respected, leading to better problem-solving and patient care (Hoare, 2023).

Incorporating actionable steps can transform these ideals into everyday practices:

Inclusion Is What We Do, Belonging Is What We Feel

- **Action versus Feeling:** Inclusion is an intentional process built into structures and processes, ensuring diverse voices are invited and valued. Belonging is the emotional outcome, where individuals feel safe, connected, and authentically part of the environment.
- **Opportunity versus Acceptance:** Inclusion creates pathways for participation, ensuring representation and access. Belonging ensures those opportunities translate into genuine acceptance, where individuals feel embraced, not just accommodated.
- **Equal Access versus Psychological Safety:** Inclusion ensures fair access to resources, spaces, and opportunities. Belonging fosters psychological safety, where individuals feel comfortable expressing themselves without fear of exclusion or judgment.
- **Journey versus Destination**: Inclusion opens doors, but belonging ensures people stay, thrive, and contribute in a meaningful way.

- **Actively solicit input** from all team members during meetings, ensuring diverse voices shape discussions.
- **Use inclusive language and practices**, affirming the value of contributions regardless of communication style or personality.
- **Encourage cross-team collaboration** to foster deeper relationships and connections among colleagues.

The dimension of Upholder in Human-Centered Leadership embodies the mindset of inclusivity and belonging. This mindset embraces the belief that every individual deserves to feel valued, heard, and empowered. It goes beyond just tolerating diversity—it actively seeks to create environments where people feel safe to contribute, be themselves, and know their presence matters.

The dimension of Upholder recognizes the unique strengths of each person and creates opportunities for them to flourish. This leader listens with empathy and curiosity to understand different perspectives and experiences. They encourage collaboration and connection, so team members feel a sense of belonging and address bias and exclusion, ensuring equity in decision-making. Most importantly, the Upholder celebrates differences and sees them as assets rather than obstacles, creating a culture of caring.

An inclusive leader doesn't just say the right things—they model intentional actions and demonstrate genuine commitment to making people feel valued. Inclusive leadership intersects with cultural competence, ensuring that belonging is nurtured across diverse healthcare environments. By recognizing cultural nuances and fostering respect, leaders empower every team member to contribute authentically. Dr. Jean Watson, in her book, *Caring Science, Mindful Practice* (2018), integrates mindfulness into leadership by emphasizing presence, intentionality, and deep human connection. Her approach fosters inclusive and authentic leadership through exhibiting a mindful presence, ensuring individuals feel truly seen, heard, and valued. She also incorporates mindfulness techniques such as self-reflection to help leaders remain grounded and intentional in their actions and decisions. According to Watson, mindfulness practice helps create and support psychologically safe spaces where individuals can thrive and flourish. Watson's Caring Science encourages leaders to lead with heart, integrating mindfulness to enhance inclusivity, authenticity, and human connection (refer to Appendix K).

When we feel a sense of true belonging, we understand that we matter; our voice and presence are influential and meaningful. In turn, we meet that basic human need to feel valued and to add value. So how do we begin to build a culture of belonging? It's all about nurturing and growing relationships. The human-centered leader as Upholder communicates a profound and meaningful message: *"I see you."* To truly see someone is to recognize their unique strengths and intrinsic value. It is through this genuine acknowledgment that we lay the foundation for a culture of caring—a culture where belonging is not just a concept, but a lived experience reflected in every interaction.

Let's go back to our meeting to put these concepts in perspective. When only inclusion exists, we may attend meetings, but we won't speak up. When belonging is present, we will engage and contribute meaningfully. When mattering is established, we know our voices shape the future of healthcare. Hospitals and healthcare systems depend on us—not just for patient care but also for the insights and leadership that drive systemic improvements. Belonging improves retention and morale. Mattering transforms passive presence into active leadership.

Human-centered leaders, as relational leaders, have the power to shift the culture from one of passive inclusion to active belonging because human-centered leaders understand the importance of mattering, both in personal and professional life. Great leadership in healthcare is not measured by how many individuals are in the room—it is measured by how many individuals know they belong, matter, and are helping shape the future of care.

Creating a Culture of Belonging

- ✓ **Use People's Names:** Personal connections start with knowing and using names. One-on-one meetings help strengthen relationships and improve name recall.
- ✓ **Begin with a Mindful Pause:** Start each meeting—including virtual ones—with a moment to recenter, refocus, and reconnect with those around you.
- ✓ **Practice Active Listening:** Foster an environment where open dialogue is encouraged and individuals feel truly heard.
- ✓ **Ensure Psychological Safety:** Create a space where people feel comfortable sharing ideas without fear of judgment.
- ✓ **Show Appreciation and Recognize Contributions:** Acknowledge and celebrate the efforts and achievements of others regularly.
- ✓ **Be Respectful:** Value diverse perspectives and maintain an atmosphere of kindness and inclusion.

Build It and They Will Come: Crafting an Environment of Belonging and Inclusion

Creating an inclusive healthcare environment starts with understanding where the organization truly stands. Tools like the Inclusivity Dial provide a clear snapshot of whether inclusivity is a genuine part of everyday operations or just an abstract goal (see Figure 10). This kind of assessment highlights gaps—whether in psychological safety, representation, or equitable access to opportunities—and brings to light both visible and hidden barriers that define the workplace culture.

From there, integrating HCD takes inclusion beyond surface-level efforts. HCD invites patients, families, and healthcare teams to co-design solutions, ensuring that inclusion becomes a tangible, lived experience. It turns policies into practice by embedding inclusivity into both the physical environment and systemic frameworks that shape day-to-day care (Norman & Verganti, 2020).

But identifying issues isn't enough—allyship transforms insights into action. Leaders have to take ownership of designing systems that prioritize equity, from rethinking who gets a seat at the decision-making table to ensuring that workflows and communication channels are intentionally inclusive. It's not just about inclusive

FIGURE 10
The Inclusivity Dial. Use this basic assessment to gauge where you feel your organization lands with Inclusion. Adapted from Frei and Morris (2020).

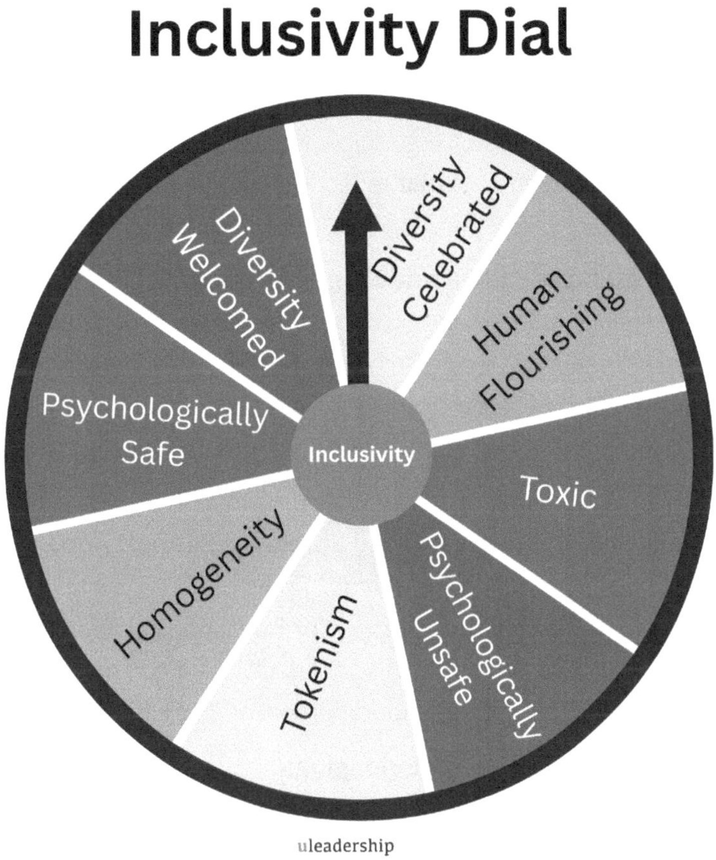

physical spaces like patient care areas or staff wellness hubs—it's about addressing the invisible frameworks too, like mentoring programs, leadership pipelines, and systems that foster psychological safety.

Ultimately, fostering inclusion isn't a one-and-done initiative. It's a cycle—a process of constant assessment, intentional design, and meaningful allyship. When healthcare leaders fully commit to this approach, inclusivity stops being a policy on paper and becomes the very foundation of workplace culture. Over time, as the Inclusivity Dial evolves, representation turns into empowerment, and healthcare systems transform into places where everyone feels seen, valued, and able to contribute to their fullest potential.

Crafting an Environment of Inclusion and Belonging—Practical Ways to Make It Happen Through Human-Centered Design (HCD)

- **Designing Inclusive Healthcare Spaces:**
  Apply HCD principles to create welcoming, accessible environments not just for patients and families, but also for healthcare employees. This includes break areas that promote well-being, ergonomic workspaces for providers, and culturally affirming design elements that reflect the diverse identities of staff and patients alike.
- **Developing Equitable Patient and Employee Portals:**
  Ensure that digital platforms empower both patients and healthcare workers by providing user-friendly access to medical records, communication tools, and wellness resources. These portals can include anonymous feedback channels for staff, allowing team members to share concerns about inclusion, psychological safety, and systemic barriers.
- **Building Inclusive Mobile Health and Employee Support Apps:**
  Design apps that meet the diverse needs of patients, caregivers, and healthcare employees, providing real-time support for both medical care and workplace well-being. This could include apps that facilitate peer mentorship, mental health support, and real-time collaboration between multidisciplinary teams.
- **Enhancing Communication for Belonging:**
  Strengthen team interactions and patient–provider relationships through inclusive language, shared decision-making models, and culturally competent communication practices. Healthcare employees need opportunities to engage in open discussions, ensuring psychological safety and trust within the workplace and during patient interactions.
- **Addressing Systemic Health Inequities and Workforce Inclusivity:**
  Leverage HCD to redesign hiring processes, leadership pipelines, and career advancement opportunities, ensuring that healthcare workers from underrepresented backgrounds feel valued and included. This involves cocreating equitable workplace policies, integrating focused training, and advocating for systemic changes that support employee well-being and professional growth.

By including healthcare employees in these initiatives, leaders ensure that inclusion and belonging permeate every layer of the organization, creating a workplace where individuals feel empowered, supported, and able to thrive.

Intentional Allyship: Designing Systems of Inclusion and Belonging in Healthcare Leadership

Allyship in healthcare leadership goes beyond just supporting inclusion—it's about intentionally creating environments where employees, patients, and families feel genuinely valued and empowered. Research shows that effective allyship means stepping into advocacy, amplifying underrepresented voices, and tackling systemic barriers head-on (Catlin, 2022). Healthcare leaders can build belonging by championing mentorship programs for historically marginalized employees, ensuring diverse representation in decision-making spaces, and fostering transparent feedback channels that allow staff to speak openly without fear of retaliation.

Allyship doesn't stop with workplace culture—it extends to patient care and community partnerships. Leaders who prioritize culturally responsive care—like providing language-accessible services, embedding trauma-informed care practices, and developing equitable hiring models—help close gaps in trust and accessibility (Nixon, 2019). A hospital executive, for instance, might collaborate with local organizations to address healthcare disparities, ensuring underserved communities receive tailored resources and support.

By embedding allyship into everyday leadership practices, healthcare organizations move past performative gestures toward lasting, systemic change. This kind of commitment benefits employees, patients, and the broader community, reshaping healthcare into a truly inclusive and empowering space.

Discussion Questions for Groups

1. How can leaders create a caring environment where everyone feels seen, heard, and valued? What are specific strategies that help foster inclusion in a team?
2. What does belonging mean in the workplace, and why is it essential for effective leadership? Can you share an example of a time when you felt a strong sense of belonging in a group or team?
3. How can you actively apply HCD principles in your daily interactions—whether as a healthcare leader, team member, patient, or community advocate—to create spaces, systems, and relationships that foster inclusion and belonging?

4. What challenges might leaders face in building an inclusive and belonging-driven culture? How can leaders overcome those obstacles to ensure everyone feels valued and engaged?

Reflection Questions for Individuals

1. How can I utilize my unique strengths to foster a more inclusive and welcoming work environment, ensuring others feel valued and supported?

____

____

____

____

____

Allyship in healthcare is most effective when it's intentional and embedded in design—not just a reactive gesture. HCD provides a framework for ensuring that allyship isn't performative, but rather woven into the structures, systems, and everyday interactions that shape inclusion and belonging. By listening to diverse perspectives, co-designing equitable solutions, and addressing systemic barriers, leaders can create workplaces and patient care environments that empower rather than exclude.

2. What intentional actions can you take as an ally to apply HCD in your workplace or community, ensuring that inclusion and belonging aren't just ideals but embedded in daily experiences?

____

____

____

____

____

References

Catlin, K. (2022). *Belonging in healthcare: The Better Allies® approach to creating more inclusive workplaces.* Better Allies Press.

Frei, F., & Morris, A. (2020). *Unleashed: The unapologetic leader's guide to empowering everyone around you.* Harvard Business Review Press.

Hoare, J. (2023). The power of connected clinical teams: From loneliness to belonging. *Philosophy, Ethics, and Humanities in Medicine, 18*(1). doi: 10.1186/s13010-023-00143-7

Nixon, S. A. (2019). The coin model of privilege and critical allyship: Implications for health. *BMC Public Health, 19,* Article 1637. doi: 10.1186/s12889-019-7884-9

Norman, D. A., & Verganti, R. (2020). Incremental and radical innovation: Design research vs. technology and meaning change. *Design Issues, 30*(1), 78–96. doi: 10.1162/DESI_a_00250

Riddle, D., & Métraux, E. (2021). Cultivating a workplace culture of belonging. *American College of Healthcare Executives.* https://www.ache.org/blog/2021/cultivating-a-workplace-culture-of-belonging

Recommended Reading

Frei, F., & Morriss, A. (2020). *Begin with trust.* Harvard Business Review Press.

Gebhardt, M. C. (2024). Editorial: Allyship—Not the solution, but a way forward. *Clinical Orthopaedics and Related Research, 482,* 217–218. doi: 10.1097/CORR.0000000000002962

CHAPTER 15

Positive Practice Environments

The Other PPE

By Christine Pabico, PhD, RN, NE-BC, FAAN, FFNMRCSI

Sr. Director, Pathway to Excellence and Well-Being Excellence American Nurses Credentialing Center

Maricon Dans, MSN, RN, NE-BC

Assistant Director, Pathway to Excellence and Well-Being Excellence Operations, American Nurses Credentialing Center

Leigh Hume, MN, RN, NE-BC

Assistant Director, Pathway to Excellence Appraisal Process, American Nurses Credentialing Center

---

If your actions inspire others to dream more, learn more, do more, and become more, you are a leader.

—John Quincy Adams

Nurses are the heartbeat of healthcare organizations, often working long hours and under immense pressure, where healthcare demands continue to stretch them to their limits. To sustain and empower this vital workforce, we must create positive practice environments, what the American Nurses Credentialing Center's (ANCC) Pathway to Excellence program considers "The Other PPE." Positive practice environments are just as essential as gloves, masks, and gowns in protecting our clinicians. Creating practice environments that foster a positive culture and center around human experience enables nurses to thrive and keep them in our profession. Pathway to Excellence (Pathway) provides an evidence-based framework with six essential standards (Shared Decision-Making, Leadership, Safety, Quality, Well-Being, and Professional Development) to do just that.

Human-Centered Design (HCD) plays a pivotal role in the enculturation of the six Pathway Standards. Its application aims to understand nurses' day-to-day experiences and motivations, address their needs and challenges, and safeguard their well-being. HCD leads to solutions that are not only effective but also empathetic and put people at the center. Human-Centered Leadership in Healthcare (HCL-HC) begins with self-awareness and radiates outward through connection, integrity, and inspiration.

Excellence by Design

By integrating HCD principles, healthcare organizations can further enhance the positive practice environments recognized by the ANCC Pathway to Excellence program.

- **Shared Decision-Making**: The first step in making nurses feel valued and heard is to listen. Gathering insight into the nurses' pain points and partnering with them to identify solutions is key. Shared decision-making becomes a powerful tool for fostering a sense of belonging, mattering, and shared purpose among team members. When team members participate in decisions, they feel like integral parts of the team, strengthening their connection to the organization. Knowing that their opinions matter boosts their motivation and engagement, as they see their input shaping the team's direction. Similarly, HCD emphasizes collaboration and co-creation, ensuring that nurses have a voice in decisions that affect their work environment. This collaborative process also aligns everyone around common goals, creating a unified vision and collective sense of purpose. This shared purpose drives engagement and commitment, making the team more cohesive and effective. The collaborative process in shared decision-making transforms the workplace into a space where everyone feels valued, connected, and motivated to achieve common goals.

- **Leadership**: Pathway emphasizes the importance of having leaders who are accessible, make their workforce a priority, and embrace their team members as integral partners in achieving unit and organizational goals. HCL-HC enables this by promoting relational leadership. As *Connectors*, they build unity in their teams through authentic communication, support, collaboration, and harnessing their team members' strengths. This is important because effective nursing leadership requires a delicate balance between the science and art of the profession. Leaders must be adept at strategic planning, ensuring that resources are allocated efficiently and operations run smoothly. However, communicating effectively and demonstrating empathy and emotional intelligence in every interaction is equally important in fostering a culture of trust and collaboration within the team. Their interpersonal skills shine through in moments of conflict resolution and patient-centered care, making everyone feel valued and heard. When leaders excel in creating a harmonious and supportive environment, both patients and staff thrive. As *Awakeners*, leaders cultivate nurses through mentoring, motivating, and advocating, unleashing their individual talents that up to this point have laid dormant in the practicalities of the nursing role. This confidence-building environment then sets the stage for leaders to serve as "architects" in creating processes that invite innovative thinking.
- **Safety**: Pathway organizations protect the psychological and physical safety of nurses and create an environment where staff feel safe expressing their ideas, concerns, errors, and discriminatory behaviors, without fear of negative consequences. HCD involves designing environments that prioritize safety and reduce risks. HCL-HC leaders create safe spaces where employees can verbalize concerns but also be a part of the solutions. The result is a positive practice environment and a culture of trust relished by nurses and patients.
- **Quality**: Pathway organizations ensure that staff are aligned with the organization's mission, vision, values, and goals. As *Connectors*, HCL-HC leaders unify their team around a shared mission and vision. Direct care nurses in Pathway organizations are involved in the review and implementation of

evidence-based practice, continuous improvement, and innovation to enhance care quality. As *Edgewalkers*, HCL-HC leaders encourage experimentation of ideas to generate innovation. The pioneering culture that results not only benefits the nurses but also leads to better patient outcomes.

- **Well-Being**: Prioritizing the physical and mental health of staff, and providing support and resources to promote well-being, is a core standard of the Pathway to Excellence. As nurses, one of the aspirations we struggle with is taking care of our own well-being. The relentless pace and emotional intensity of the job often leave little room for self-care, leading to burnout and stress. We also know that "no one can drink from an empty cup." Leaders who embody the principles of HCL-HC prioritize self-care for themselves to set the tone for everyone and be a beacon for their team. *Self* as a leadership dimension puts well-being, self-care, self-compassion, self-awareness, and mindfulness as priorities in leading teams. When leaders practice self-care, they can provide the support their team needs, their empathy shines through in every interaction, and they create a safe space for proactively taking steps toward maintaining their well-being. More important is the powerful message and example they set for their team members. They understand that by taking care of their own well-being, it essentially gives their team members "permission" to do the same. This approach fosters a culture where self-care is valued and encouraged, helping to mitigate burnout and improve overall job satisfaction, fulfillment, and engagement, which leads to nurses providing higher quality care. Leaders as the *Upholder* are also emotionally, socially, organizationally aware, and personally well and healthy. The result is an exceptional experience for nurses and patients, which reflects a culture of care.
- **Professional Development**: Pathway organizations value and recognize the importance of lifelong learning, ongoing education, specialty certification, and professional development. Education on respectful communication is also included to ensure a positive and professional work environment. Leaders who embrace HCD principles create safe spaces for respectful communication. By fostering a culture of respect and continuous learning, HCL-HC leaders seek to *Awaken* the potential in their team members, often beyond what they see in themselves. HCL-HC leaders coach, mentor, and advocate for individual team members' professional growth because they know individual success transforms into organizational success. They support ongoing learning and development, ensuring that nurses have opportunities for growth and mentorship.

Great leaders don't just lead—they create spaces where people feel seen, heard, and valued. Under their guidance, you don't just work—you belong.

Beyond the Blueprint: Bringing Pathway to Life

Dr. Kevin K. McEwan, DNP, RN, NEA-BC, FAONL Chief Nursing Officer at Madison Health, often shares,

"The Pathway framework is the secret recipe!"

During the height of the COVID-19 pandemic, when healthcare systems were under immense strain, Kevin didn't just lead; he relied on the Pathway to Excellence framework as a sound foundation to navigate through the challenges. In doing so, he embodies the essence of HCL-HC, a philosophy grounded in authenticity, empathy, and purpose. According to Kevin, Human-Centered Leadership (HCL) starts with him being aware of himself, being present, and dedicated to his own personal growth. He acts purposefully, modeling calm, clarity, and compassion in the midst of ambiguity. His leadership does not revolve around control, but rather around relationships and connections. Kevin integrates these practices into his daily interactions, which are fundamental manifestations of the HCL traits, such as empathy, empowerment, collaboration, and ethical leadership, proving to be a clear testimony to his commitment to nurturing a healthy and inclusive organizational culture.

As a **Connector**, Kevin cultivates a culture of **Shared Decision-Making**, ensuring that nurses and interprofessional teams have a voice in driving their own practice. Through daily rounding, open dialogue, and inclusive team huddles, he has fostered a culture of trust and teamwork where every voice is valued and every contribution is appreciated. Kevin empowers his team to drive initiatives and lead meaningful changes, fostering positive cultures where nurses feel respected, heard, and recognized.

A powerful example of Kevin's leadership style emerged when he recognized that a seasoned nurse, often regarded as an informal leader, was experiencing burnout and feeling unheard. In response, he engaged her to co-chair the newly established facility-wide shared governance council. Through a combination of internal professional governance training and participation in a national conference, she began to flourish in her role, later sharing, "I have never felt this engaged in my career." Although her term at the facility Nurse Practice Council has since ended, she has remained a vocal and influential informal leader within her department, now sitting as chair of the unit-based council. She nurtures her engagement, reinvigorating her passion for nursing and enhancing her career. She embraces her role as a catalyst for positive change, an outcome made possible by Kevin's unwavering support and belief in her potential.

As an **Upholder**, Kevin exemplifies the **Leadership** standard, leading with integrity, consistency, and transparency. He sets a strong ethical tone, advocates for both staff and patients, and creates a psychologically safe environment where people feel supported, respected, and valued, which extends to the patients. His actions reinforce a culture built on trust, inclusion, and accountability. Kevin's vision is to achieve cultural excellence that benefits all staff and patients, including international clients and their respective families. This vision was well exemplified when they got bestowed the DAISY recognition, with their story amplified on several occasions and various platforms.

As an **Awakener**, Kevin inspires his team with a compelling vision of what healthcare should look like within the four walls of their organization, nurturing excellence in his team even in the most uncertain times. He brings the **Safety** standard to life, encompassing not only physical safety but also emotional and psychological safety in a holistic manner. His gentle approach to motivating and guiding others through setbacks has awakened a renewed sense of meaning and purpose. This was especially exemplified when one of his units received compelling DAISY recognition from a couple from the United Kingdom.

Kevin fosters **Well-Being**, recognizing that caregiver wellness is essential to delivering exceptional care. Under his leadership, access to mental health resources, wellness programs, and resilience-building strategies expanded. He modeled work–life balance and encouraged others to prioritize their own well-being and care for their individual families, fostering a culture of caring where people could thrive.

Kevin championed **Professional Development**, encouraging bold thinking, continuous learning, and leadership growth. He has mentored emerging leaders, even beyond the walls of his organization, through his partnership with the American Organization of Nurse Leaders. He selflessly devotes his time to mentoring, particularly in rural healthcare settings. He celebrated certifications and supported career advancement, aligning with the standard that promotes lifelong learning and professional excellence. One compelling example of the Clinical Ladder Program's impact highlights how it has inspired nurses to elevate their clinical expertise through exploring specialty certification. At the outset of Madison Health's Pathway to Excellence journey and the launch of the Clinical Ladder Program, fewer than ten nurses held professional certifications. However, by fostering a culture of empowerment, encouraging nurses to take ownership of their professional growth, and leveraging the organization's partnership with the Success Pays program, remarkable progress has been achieved. In just four years, Madison Health has nearly quadrupled its number of certified nurses, with many attaining multiple certifications to deepen their expertise and enhance the quality of care provided. One nurse holds three certifications in medical–surgical nursing and ostomy care. As the only certified ostomy nurse in her region of Iowa, she is a vital resource for both providers and patients, consistently supporting the complex and specialized needs of those affected. She credits the organization's investment in her professional development as a key contributor to her "sense of accomplishment and well-being."

And through it all, he reinforces the **Quality** standard, ensuring that every decision and initiative is aligned with his vision, providing the utmost standards of care and excellence in nursing practice. His strategic foresight and commitment to positive outcomes reflected a deep dedication to his constant pursuit of excellence.

The impact of this leadership was powerfully illustrated when several nurses who had left Madison Health, Idaho, to pursue travel nursing subsequently decided to return. When asked what brought them back, their response was simple yet profound.

"This is our home, Kevin. This is where we belong."

The nurses' words reflect more than mere appreciation; they speak to a culture of belonging, trust, and human connection brought about by Kevin's integration of HCL and the Pathway framework. By leading with compassion, integrity, and shared vision, Kevin didn't just navigate a crisis; he cultivated a thriving, purpose-driven community of nurses who feel empowered to stay, grow, and then THRIVE.

At Atrium Health Navicent Peach, the journey to becoming a Pathway to Excellence-designated hospital has been one of transformation, collaboration, and resolute commitment to the community. At the heart of this achievement is Jill Hancock, MSN, RN, OCN, Chief Nursing Officer—a human-centered leader whose passion, vision, and presence have not only guided the pursuit of this prestigious designation but also have redefined what it means to lead with purpose.

From the moment Jill accepted the challenge to lead the Pathway journey, she brought more than just expertise—she brought the heart.

Jill's leadership, grounded in the Pathway to Excellence framework, is a living example of HCL. Jill led with presence, humility, and authenticity. She demonstrates emotional intelligence and resilience, consistently showing up for her team, especially during challenging times. It is not a surprise that she became a recipient of the Pathway Nurse of the Year Award for Nursing Leadership, presented by ANCC, recognizing Jill as an outstanding nurse leader who has made a profound impact on their practice environment, exemplifying transformational leadership by inspiring and influencing her teams across departments, fostering shared governance, and ensuring that her team's voices are heard. Recipients of this award are recognized for their creative problem-solving skills, hands-on leadership style, and ability to foster strong, trust-based relationships with their teams. Her leadership had a positive impact on various organizational outcomes, including enhanced staff engagement, reduced turnover, and improved patient care quality.

As a **Connector**, Jill fosters **Shared Decision-Making**, ensuring that nurses and interprofessional teams are not only included in organizational decisions but also empowered to lead such initiatives. Her leadership is deeply relational, always exemplified, whether she's rounding with her snack cart or stepping in to help with patient care, Jill is present and engaged. One powerful example of her servant leadership occurred when she personally helped bathe a patient in the seclusion room of the emergency room, where she gently combed the mats from the patient's hair. This profound act of compassion reflects her philosophy that no task is beneath her and that every person deserves dignity and utmost care.

As an **Upholder**, Jill lives the **Leadership** standard, leading with unwavering integrity and commitment. Jill's commitment to health equity and community engagement reflected her deeply rooted values and belief in always doing what is right. Under her leadership, Atrium Health Navicent Peach eliminated contract labor and achieved a 0% vacancy rate after embarking on the Pathway journey. She also led the hospital to become the first Pathway-designated facility in the Advocate Health system, a milestone celebrated with nurses and her entire healthcare team in joyful unity. With her exemplary leadership, the Pathway journey yielded remarkable outcomes that include nursing vacancy rates dropping from 30% to 0%, patient satisfaction scores increasing from 64% to 81%, and quality outcomes exceeding expectations across the board. Jill's leadership not only aligned with the Pathway Standards but also exemplified the core values of HCL-HC by cultivating trust, teamwork, and a deep sense of purpose among her team.

As an **Awakener**, Jill inspires her team to pursue excellence in healthcare at all costs, living by the Pathway Standards. Her ability to guide and motivate others amid turmoil has provided a sense of deeper purpose for nursing practice within her organization. She mentored emerging leaders, celebrated certifications, and supported career advancements and growth. One nurse shared how Jill trained her for a nurse manager role, mentored her growth, and even prayed with her during a personal loss—an act of compassion that has left a lasting impact. It is no wonder that the emergency room manager once mentioned, "She is literally the best human being I know!"

She also prioritizes **Well-Being** by role-modeling behaviors and recognizing that caregiver wellness is essential to delivering exceptional care. She implemented strategies to foster the well-being of her teams, spearheading the securing of grants for a snack cart and a Zen Den, modeling work–life balance, and encouraging others to care for themselves, thereby fostering a culture of health that enabled her team to thrive. Additionally, Jill is a driving force behind **Professional Development**, inspiring bold thinking, fostering a culture of continuous learning, and nurturing the next generation of leaders. She actively mentored emerging nurse leaders, celebrated professional milestones such as certifications, and advocated for career advancement, aligning with the standard that values lifelong learning and the continuous pursuit of excellence. Throughout her leadership, Jill remains steadfast in upholding the **Quality** Standard. She ensured that every initiative, decision, and innovation was rooted in the highest principles of patient care and nursing practice. Her firm commitment and dedication cultivated a culture where excellence wasn't just encouraged, it was an expected norm. Under her guidance, innovation flourished, accountability was embraced, and compassion remained at the heart of every nursing endeavor.

The impact of Jill's leadership is deeply felt. She inspires teammates to pursue higher education, supports career advancement, and celebrates every success—big or small. Her dedication to servant leadership, her steadfast belief in the team, and her relentless pursuit of excellence have created a ripple effect that will be felt for years to come.

One of the nurses so aptly describes her:

> "Jill Hancock is more than a leader—she is a catalyst for change, a champion of people, and a living embodiment of the Pathway to Excellence vision. Her legacy is one of compassion, courage, and commitment to a future where every caregiver is empowered, every voice is valued, and every patient receives the highest standard of care."

Another nurse leader adds, *"She is the type of leader you want to role model yourself after. She genuinely cares about those she works with, and it shows."*

The Best Place to Start: Look in the Mirror!

Pathway to Excellence is not simply a strategy—it's a culture; it provides a framework that sustains an environment where nurses feel heard, respected, and valued. HCL is about leading with the heart and shifting focus from protocols and task completion to empathy and advocacy.

The seamless integration of the four dimensions of HCL-HC (Self, Awakener, Connector, and Upholder) into the Pathway framework (Shared Decision-Making, Leadership, Safety, Quality, Well-Being, and Professional Development) transforms the work environment from operational to fundamentally human where nurses no longer just survive; they belong, grow, matter, and *thrive*.

A starting point for organizations embarking on the Pathway journey is to conduct a self-assessment to determine where gaps in the framework exist within their organization. Leaders can take this same approach of assessing their own strengths and opportunities when learning to lead with the heart. Just as Kevin recognized that HCL starts with self-awareness, all leaders are encouraged to embark on their own journey of self-reflection.

Consider how you would answer the questions below. And more importantly, consider whether your nurses would agree with your response.

When reflecting on your own leadership style, do you:	Y/N	Strategies to strengthen "leading with the heart."
• Foster a culture of belonging that makes each team member feel they matter?		
• Create an environment where your nurses feel like their contributions are valued?		
• Dedicate time with each nurse to better understand their strengths and what they enjoy most about their day-to-day work? • Advocate for opportunities that allow them to build upon their strengths and foster what they enjoy doing? • Provide a process that invites innovative thinking?		
• Create safe spaces for open dialogue to actively address concerns that negatively impact their psychological and physical safety? • Listen to understand versus listen to respond?		
• Think your nurses trust that you will follow up on those concerns?		

- Align your nurses with the mission and vision of the organization?
- Encourage collaborative efforts in continuous improvement initiatives?

- Place well-being as a priority through modeling self-care?
- Foster mental and physical health practices that reduce burnout?
- Ask your nurses for ideas on what activities or support during the workday would benefit their mental health and well-being?
- Engage your nurses in discussions on whether they feel the strategies put in place to enhance their mental health and well-being are making a difference?

- Encourage and support lifelong learning through education and mentoring opportunities that promote personal growth?

Final Thoughts

The art and science of leadership encompasses a blend of strategic thinking and emotional intelligence. While technical skills and strategic acumen are vital, it is the soft skills—such as empathy, communication, and authenticity—that truly inspire and motivate team members. These essential skills foster trust, collaboration, and a sense of belonging, enabling leaders to connect with their teams on a deeper level. By prioritizing these human-centered qualities, leaders can cultivate an environment where individuals feel valued and empowered, ultimately driving collective success and innovation. When leaders focus on building a culture of engagement and connection, nurses flourish and see a powerful reason to stay.

Discussion Question for Groups

How can HCL-HC and HCD be leveraged to create Positive Practice Environments that support nurses' well-being and professional fulfillment? Consider how the six Pathway Standards—Shared Decision-Making, Leadership, Safety, Quality, Well-Being, and Professional Development—can be strengthened through leadership approaches that prioritize psychological safety, empathy, and inclusion.

Reflection Questions for Individuals

Reflect on a time when a workplace environment either supported or hindered your ability to thrive as a nurse. How might the principles of HCL and HCD have improved the culture, strengthened team collaboration, or safeguarded well-being? What lessons can be applied to creating a more sustainable and fulfilling nursing practice?

____

____

____

____

____

Recommended Reading

Barnes, B., Barnes, M., & Pabico, C. (2021). Meaningful recognition: An imperative for nurse well-being. *Nursing Management (Springhouse), 52*(10), 6–9. doi: 10.1097/01.NUMA.0000792044.13706.b2

Bates, M., Pabico, C., Dans, M., & Hume, L. (2024). 2024 Pathway manual introduction. *Nursing Management (Springhouse), 55*(4), 6–10. doi: 10.1097/nmg.0000000000000113

Grant, E. J., & Pabico, C. (2022). A framework for achieving the National Plan for Health Workforce Well-Being recommendations. *Nursing Management (Springhouse), 53*(10), 9–15. doi: 10.1097/01.NUMA.0000874432.64403.fb

Leclerc, L., & Pabico, C. (2023). Blueprints for well-being: Modeling the way through Human-Centered Leadership and Pathway to Excellence. *Nursing Management (Springhouse), 54*(4), 9–16. doi: 10.1097/01.NUMA.0000921892.27917.78

Human-Centered Understanding

Human-Centered Understanding cultivates trust, accountability, and possibility-driven leadership. *Appreciative inquiry* shifts focus from problems to strengths, empowering individuals and teams to envision and create meaningful change. *Just culture* reinforces psychological safety by balancing accountability with learning, ensuring errors are addressed constructively rather than punitively. Together with HCL-HC, these principles create an environment where openness, fairness, and growth lead to stronger collaboration, innovation, and shared understanding in healthcare settings.

CHAPTER 16

Appreciative Inquiry

Building on Strengths to Design the Future

"The best way to predict the future is to create it."

—Peter Drucker

Imagine a way to create change that doesn't start by fixing what's wrong but by building on what's strong. Appreciative inquiry offers a fresh perspective—a possibility-focused approach that energizes teams and organizations by tapping into their collective strengths and aspirations. It's a shift from problem-solving to possibility-creating, emphasizing the positive elements that inspire growth and transformation. If you've ever wondered how to spark meaningful, lasting change while empowering the people at the heart of it, appreciative inquiry might just be the approach you've been looking for. Let's explore how this powerful method works and why it's redefining what change can truly mean.

Appreciative inquiry is a way to create solutions that truly reflect the needs and strengths of the people involved. It's all about empowering those on the frontlines—the ones who really understand the work—to come together and make positive changes in their environment. Instead of focusing on problems, appreciative inquiry highlights possibilities, looking at what drives energy and success while appreciating the unique talents each team member brings.

At its core, appreciative inquiry is a team effort, relying on collaboration and participation. By tapping into everyone's ideas, experiences, and diverse perspectives, the group creates a shared vision that drives meaningful change. Since the solutions come directly from the people doing the work, they feel a sense of ownership and accountability for the results. This equal and inclusive process makes the change more effective and lasting.

Core Principles of Appreciative Inquiry

Appreciative inquiry is a powerful approach that helps teams transform their aspirations into meaningful, actionable change. Rooted in a human-centered philosophy, appreciative inquiry is built on five key principles identified in seminal work by renowned appreciative inquiry expert and original theorist, Dr. David Cooperrider (Cooperrider & Srivastva, 1987; Cooperrider & Whitney, 2005):

- **The Constructionist Principle**: Meaningful change begins with the people at the heart of an organization. The way we understand and shape our experiences influences how we grow and evolve together.
- **The Simultaneity Principle**: Change starts the moment we ask a question. Inquiry and action are deeply connected, sparking momentum from the very first conversation.
- **The Poetic Principle**: Stories shape our shared reality. As teams and individuals evolve, so do the narratives that inspire and guide them toward the future.
- **The Anticipatory Principle**: Imagination fuels transformation. A team's vision of what's possible serves as a driving force in creating a better future.
- **The Positivity Principle**: Strength-based approaches foster deeper connections and sustainable change. By focusing on what works and aligning around shared goals, organizations cultivate lasting impact.

Together, these principles celebrate the collective human experience, making appreciative inquiry a valuable tool for leaders who want to create meaningful, lasting change.

Show Me the Evidence!

For over 30 years, appreciative inquiry has been a powerful tool for driving meaningful change in healthcare, offering a positive and possibility-focused approach to change. Its applications range from evaluating and *improving organizational and clinical processes* (Fernald, Smyrnios, & Vitello, 2020; Jesus et al., 2024; Martinez, 2017; Merriel et al., 2022; Richer, Ritchie, & Marchionni, 2010; Trajkovski, Schmied, Vickers, & Jackson, 2013) to *fostering professional growth and identity development* (Best, Robbé, & Williams, 2022; Hung et al., 2018). By *enhancing the quality of care* (Fernald et al., 2020; Jesus et al., 2024; Regula & Gobbens, 2023) and *helping teams create unified visions* (Best et al., 2022), appreciative inquiry has contributed to more collaborative and impactful healthcare environments. Additionally, it has played a role in *improving workplace dynamics* (Best et al., 2022; Merriel et al., 2022; Regula & Gobbens, 2023; Trajkovski et al., 2013) and *bridging the gap between research and practice in hospital settings* (Hung et al., 2018; Merriel et al., 2022). Appreciative inquiry's ability to inspire and drive change demonstrates its value as a strategic framework in advancing healthcare systems. It provides a foundation for envisioning what's possible and turning those aspirations into tangible progress.

Using the Appreciative Inquiry Model to Transform Nursing Practice

In 2022, we published an article on how to use the appreciative inquiry process to engage nurses in making changes in nursing practice (Kennedy, Leclerc, & Campis, 2022). Here's how we applied the 4D process.

Discover

The first step is defining the focus for the inquiry and identifying what works well. A leader can play a key role in establishing this focus, ensuring the team begins with a shared understanding. This phase centers on open conversations that highlight strengths—exploring "what is currently working well" and "what has worked well in the past."

Team members are encouraged to share stories of meaningful moments that foster positive connections and uplifting memories. Thoughtful questions guide the discussion, such as: *What brings you joy at work? What do you appreciate about your current practice model? When have you felt valued by colleagues, patients, families, or the organization?*

These conversations help uncover alignment between personal, professional, and organizational values, allowing patterns and themes to emerge. A facilitator and researcher can support the process, helping the team emphasize strengths and build on them as the foundation for transformation. This phase is about fostering a positive mindset and setting the stage for meaningful change.

Dream

This step focuses on creativity and imagination, inspiring teams to envision possibilities for the future. Questions designed to spark engagement might include: *What would nursing practice look like if transformed overnight? If you could wave a magic wand, what would the ideal work environment feel like and achieve?*

All ideas are welcomed during brainstorming, with guidance to keep the team centered on opportunities rather than challenges or obstacles. This process generates creative concepts that can shape a shared vision for the future, paving the way for the next phase of action.

Design

The design phase brings the team's vision into focus and builds a clear path forward. It's about turning ideas into actionable plans for the future. Questions might include: *What should nurse practice in the organization be known for? How does each team member contribute to the broader vision? What support is needed for the interprofessional team to excel?*

These discussions lead to *provocative propositions*—forward-thinking statements that articulate the ideal state of practice as though it's already achieved. Facilitators and researchers help refine these ideas into a practical framework, aligning the team's aspirations with actionable steps to bring them to life.

Deliver

The final phase focuses on implementation, with teams developing detailed action plans for each strategic goal. Collaboration is crucial, as interprofessional teams work together to ensure alignment and shared ownership of the change process.

During this stage, teams may integrate structured methods such as Plan, Do, Study, Act; Lean Management; or Six Sigma to bring about sustainable improvement. The goal is to embed the changes into standard practice by following both process and outcome metrics.

Strong leadership is essential, with designated leaders guiding each part of the plan. A trained facilitator and project manager provide the necessary support to keep efforts organized and moving toward success. While this phase requires time and dedication, it ensures meaningful transformation that is grounded in collaboration and evidence-based methods (Kennedy et al., 2022).

Appreciative inquiry, shaped by the Human-Centered Leadership in Healthcare framework in Figure 11, is all about using what's already working to drive meaningful

FIGURE 11

Appreciative Inquiry: The Human-Centered Way. This model illustrates the appreciative inquiry 4D process with the Human-Centered Leadership in Healthcare dimensions superimposed indicating the compatibility.

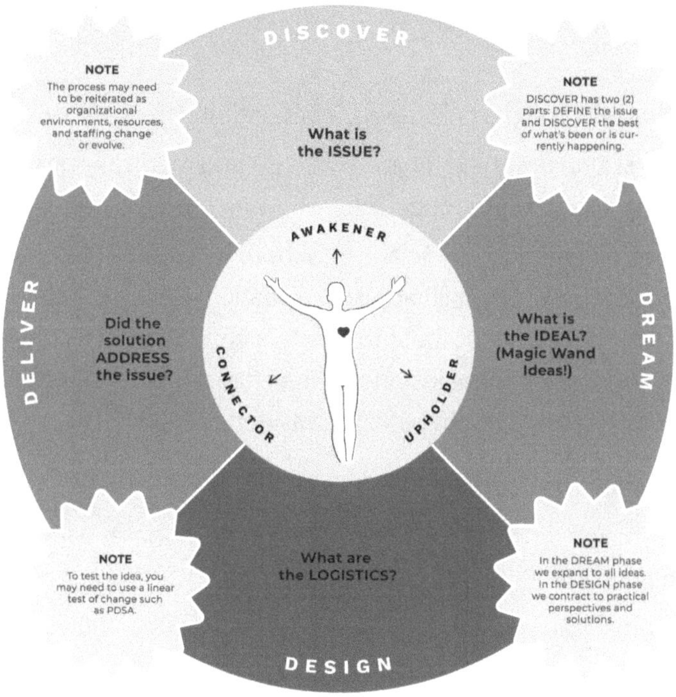

change. Instead of getting stuck on problems, it helps teams focus on strengths, build trust, and create solutions together. Let's take a look at an all too common, real-world problem: patient handover from the emergency department (ED) to a medical–surgical unit. When appreciative inquiry is applied to the patient handoff process, this approach helps staff reimagine how transitions can be smoother, safer, more efficient, and centered around teamwork.

Appreciative Inquiry Unleashed!

The uLeadership team has successfully used the appreciative inquiry process to collaborate with groups across the country. Together, interprofessional teams have created change processes that address important issues such as organizational values and purpose, team building, trust, well-being, professional identity, and psychological safety. There are key practices that have proven essential for success: fostering a

CASE EXAMPLE

Improving the Patient Handoff Process from Emergency Department to a Medical–Surgical Unit

Discovering Our Strengths

- **Goal:** Identify current strengths in the ED-to-medical–surgical unit handoff process.
- **Question:** What aspects of the patient handoff process are working well?
- **Activities:** One-on-one interviews with ED and medical–surgical nurses, interdisciplinary focus groups, and reviewing past successful handoffs.
- **Example:** Nurses and physicians from both units recognize that structured communication tools, such as SBAR (Situation–Background–Assessment–Recommendation), contribute to effective handoffs when consistently used. They also highlight instances where teamwork and proactive coordination have led to smooth patient transitions.

Dreaming for the Future

- **Goal:** Envision an ideal handoff process that eliminates gaps and promotes continuity of care.
- **Question:** What would an optimized patient handoff process look like?
- **Activities:** Large-group brainstorming, vision mapping, and storytelling exercises to describe an ideal scenario.
- **Example:** A medical–surgical nurse imagines a system where real-time digital updates flow seamlessly between departments, eliminating missing or delayed information. Another team member envisions a dedicated transition nurse who ensures that both teams are fully aligned before patient transfer.

Designing Our Future

- **Goal:** Identify strategic priorities that bring the dream to life.
- **Question:** What top priorities will move us toward an improved handoff process?
- **Activities:** Ranking improvement ideas using multivoting, creating a roadmap with timelines and action items, and defining accountability structures. Integrate recent evidence to support the interventions.

CASE EXAMPLE

- **Example:** Staff propose integrating a standardized electronic handoff tool, incorporating checklists to verify completion of key steps, and scheduling brief interdisciplinary huddles before patient transfers.

Delivering the Solution

- **Goal:** Implement actionable strategies to enhance the handoff process.
- **Activities:** Small group planning sessions, stakeholder collaborations, setting measurable success indicators, outlining follow-up evaluations. Perform iterative Plan, Do, Study, Act processes to test the ideas.
- **Example:** The team pilots a streamlined electronic communication tool for handoff documentation, launching training sessions for staff across both units. Monthly check-ins assess improvements, and a recognition system is established to celebrate teams that demonstrate excellence in patient transitions.

psychologically safe environment where individuals feel comfortable sharing ideas, ensuring shared ownership of the process, and celebrating short-term successes to keep the momentum going. By focusing on these principles, teams are empowered to take full ownership of both the change process and its outcomes, creating meaningful and lasting transformation.

Change doesn't have to feel overwhelming or out of control. Appreciative inquiry transforms change into an uplifting and empowering experience, where ideas thrive, strengths shine, and progress unfolds. It invites leaders and teams to focus on what's working, imagine what's possible, and build a collaborative path toward their desired future.

Discussion Questions for Groups

1. What is one change your team could help shape to create a better future for your unit or department?
2. Which change management process does your organization use most often? Is it a process that could complement appreciative inquiry in the deliver phase?

3. How might focusing on your team's strengths and successes spark new possibilities for growth and innovation within your unit or department?

Reflection for Individuals

Consider the appreciative inquiry process—discover, dream, design, and deliver. How does this approach align with your leadership style? Do you tend to focus on problems and deficits? Are you quick to offer your own solutions? Or do you build on what's working well, empowering your team to innovate and lead the decision-making process?

____

____

____

____

____

References

Best, S., Robbé, I., & Williams, S. (2022). Mobilizing professional identity in multidisciplinary teams: An appreciative inquiry. *International Journal of Healthcare Management, 15*(2), 132–141.

Cooperrider, D. L., & Srivastva, S. (1987). Appreciative inquiry in organizational life. In R. W. Woodman & W. A. Pasmore (Eds.), *Research in organizational change and development* (Vol. 1, pp. 129–169). JAI Press.

Cooperrider, D. L., & Whitney, D. (2005). *Appreciative inquiry: A positive revolution in change.* Berrett-Koehler.

Fernald, M. M., Smyrnios, N. A., & Vitello, J. (2020). Early mobility for critically ill patients: Building staff commitment through appreciative inquiry. *Critical Care Nurse, 40*(4), 66–72.

Hung, L., Phinney, A., Chaudhury, H., Rodney, P., Tabamo, J., & Bohl, D. (2018). Appreciative inquiry: Bridging research and practice in a hospital setting. *International Journal of Qualitative Methods, 17*, 1–10.

Jesus, T. S., Buschbacher, J., Struhar, J., Walters, T., Lopez, C., Fernandez, A., . . . Colby, K. (2024). What is so great about inpatient rehabilitation from the patient experience perspective: Qualitative content analysis of an appreciative inquiry during a bedside experience rounding. *Healthcare, 12*(17), 1711.

Kennedy, K., Leclerc, L., & Campis, S. (2022). The great realization: Nurses are in the driver's seat. *Nurse Leader, 20*(5), 480–484.

Martinez, H. (2017). *The integration of visuals and appreciative inquiry for organizational change.* Retrieved from https://www.centerforappreciativeinquiry.net/wp-content/uploads/2018/01/AI_CaseStudyExamples_HeatherMartinez_20170212.pdf

Merriel, A., Wilson, A., Decker, E., Hussein, J., Larkin, M., Barnard, K., O'Dair, M., Costello, A., Malata, A., & Coomarasamy, A. (2022). Systematic review and narrative synthesis of the impact of appreciative inquiry in healthcare. *BMJ Open Quality, 11,* Article e001911. doi: 10.1136/bmjoq-2022-001911

Regula, V. G., & Gobbens, R. J. (2023). Learning and developing together for improving the quality of care in a nursing home, is appreciative inquiry the key? *Healthcare, 11*(13), 1840.

Richer, M. C., Ritchie, J., & Marchionni, C. (2010). Appreciative inquiry in healthcare. *British Journal of Healthcare Management, 16*(4), 164–172.

Trajkovski, S., Schmied, V., Vickers, M., & Jackson, D. (2013). Implementing the 4D cycle of appreciative inquiry in health care: A methodological review. *Journal of Advanced Nursing, 69*(6), 1224–1234.

Recommended Reading

Achor, S. (2018). *The happiness advantage: How a positive brain fuels success in work and Life.* Crown Currency.

Cooperrider, D. L., Sorensen, P. F., Jr., Yaeger, T. F., & Whitney, D. (2001). *Appreciative inquiry: An emerging direction for organization development.* Stipes Publishing.

Cooperrider, D. L., Whitney, D., & Stavros, J. M. (2003). *Appreciative inquiry handbook.* Lakeshore Publisher.

Smith, A. (2023). *Practical appreciative inquiry: How to use this leading-edge coaching method confidently with teams and small groups.* Coaching Leaders.

Stavros, J., & Torres, C. (2021). *Conversations worth having, second edition: Using appreciative inquiry to fuel productive and meaningful engagement.* Berrett-Koehler.

CHAPTER 17

Just Culture

The Pillar of Psychological Safety

The only real mistake is the one from which we learn nothing.

—Henry Ford, American industrialist

Have you ever hesitated before speaking up about an error or concern in your workplace? That pause—the fear of judgment, retaliation, or blame—is exactly why just culture matters. In healthcare, mistakes happen, not because people are careless, but because systems aren't perfect and we're humans who make honest mistakes. Yet, too often, errors are met with finger-pointing instead of learning and prevention. Just culture flips the script by creating psychologically safe environments, where healthcare professionals feel empowered to report issues without fear of punishment.

Think of just culture like a safety net, not to excuse recklessness but to separate honest mistakes from negligence. Research shows that when organizations focus on fixing system flaws rather than blaming individuals, error reporting increases, patient outcomes improve, and teams work with more confidence (Välimäki, Johnson, & Lee, 2024). It's the difference between silencing voices and amplifying them—which directly impacts safety, trust, and quality of care (van Baarle et al., 2022).

Now, let's connect this to Human-Centered Leadership in Healthcare (HCL-HC) because just culture doesn't exist without strong leadership backing it up. Leaders set the tone for how errors and concerns are handled. Are mistakes treated as opportunities for growth, or are they met with fear and retribution? Human-centered leaders understand that trust and transparency aren't just buzzwords—they are the backbone of ethical accountability (American Nurses Association, 2024). When leaders model fairness, open communication, and system-based problem-solving, they create a workplace where nurses, physicians, and staff feel safe to speak up and innovate (Murray, Clifford, Larson, Lee, & Sculli, 2023). And that's not just good for morale, it's critical for patient safety.

Psychological safety isn't a luxury, it's a necessity. Teams that feel safe to admit mistakes, share ideas, and ask questions are the ones driving real innovation and improvement in healthcare. Imagine an environment where people aren't afraid to speak up, where concerns are met with collaboration, not punishment (Lansing et al., 2023). That's the power of Just Culture. And for healthcare leaders, the question isn't "Should we implement it?"—it's "How fast can we get started?"

Psychological Safety: Removing Fear to Encourage Transparency

Imagine working in a healthcare environment where you feel completely safe to speak up whether it's reporting an error, voicing a concern, or offering a new idea. That's the essence of psychological safety—a culture built on trust, transparency, and open communication. When teams feel empowered to share openly without fear of punishment or retaliation, collaboration deepens, innovation flourishes, and patient care improves (Välimäki et al., 2024). But the flip side? In fear-based workplaces, mistakes get buried instead of addressed, burnout rises, and staff withdraw instead of engage. And in healthcare, where split-second decisions impact lives, silence can be dangerous. The real question isn't "Should we prioritize psychological safety?"—it's "How do we make it happen?" The answer? Leadership—specifically, the Connector dimension of Human-Centered Leadership (HCL), where leaders cultivate trust, create safe spaces for honest conversations, and model openness in every interaction.

Connectors are leaders who cultivate trust by making vulnerability and openness a norm. They create environments where nurses and healthcare professionals feel valued, heard, and safe to express concerns without fear of retribution. Consider the experience of Emily, a new intensive care unit (ICU) nurse, who was working under a punitive leadership model. One night, during a high-pressure shift, she realized that she missed giving a scheduled dose of an antibiotic for a sepsis patient. Immediately realizing her mistake, she was terrified to report it, fearing backlash and disciplinary action. A senior nurse advised her to stay quiet, warning her that reporting could lead to an incident report that might harm her career. Out of fear, Emily hesitated, choosing silence over transparency. Now, compare this scenario to a just culture approach—led by a Connector, who nurtures a climate of trust and learning. In this case, Emily's mistake would have led to an open conversation with leadership, allowing her team to review workflow challenges together and improve processes systemwide rather than focusing on individual blame (Lesandrini & Leclerc, 2024; Murray et al., 2023). Instead of punishing errors, a Connector leads with curiosity, asking: *"How can we design a system that helps prevent this from happening again?"*

The consequences of a fear-based culture are far-reaching. Underreporting leads to repeated errors, burnout skyrockets as staff carry unspoken stress, and disengagement becomes inevitable. When nurses feel unsupported or afraid to report mistakes, they withdraw from proactive problem-solving, leading to less collaboration and poorer patient outcomes (Elmi et al., 2025). Connectors disrupt this cycle by prioritizing relational trust and psychological safety. They encourage teams to ask questions, challenge assumptions, and share insights freely, fostering open communication and shared accountability. Healthcare teams led by Connectors don't just perform better—they feel better, creating an environment where people flourish rather than simply endure.

The key takeaway? Psychological safety isn't about eliminating accountability—it's about transforming it. A just culture led by a Connector ensures that mistakes are learning moments rather than career-ending incidents, reinforcing trust and systemwide improvement. Healthcare leaders must commit to fostering psychological safety, not just through policy—but through consistent, relational leadership. By embracing open dialogue, fair accountability, and ethical decision-making, organizations can protect both their staff and their patients, leading to a safer, more resilient healthcare system.

Error Management—From Individual Blame to Systemic Learning

Mistakes happen in healthcare not because nurses or clinicians are careless, but because systems aren't perfect and human error is bound to happen. The traditional approach to errors has often focused on individual blame, creating a culture where staff fear reporting mistakes instead of learning from them. Just culture shifts this mindset, recognizing that most errors result from systemwide issues rather than personal failures (Välimäki et al., 2024). Instead of punishing individuals for making mistakes, just culture identifies patterns, examines workflows, and strengthens processes to prevent recurrence. Accountability doesn't mean punishment—it means creating an environment where errors lead to improvements, not fear.

Let's revisit Emily, the ICU nurse who hesitated to report her medication omission due to fear of backlash. Under a punitive system, she might have been reprimanded or faced professional consequences, discouraging her from speaking up in the future. But what if her hospital embraced Just Culture, led by a socially and organizationally aware leader—an Upholder? In this environment, the error wouldn't be treated as an isolated mistake but as a potential systemwide issue. Upon review, leadership might discover staffing shortages, unclear protocols, or inefficient electronic health record processes contributed to the omission. Rather than placing the blame solely on Emily, the focus would shift to how the organization could refine workflows to prevent similar errors. This approach reinforces trust, fairness, and collective accountability which are hallmarks of HCL (Leclerc, Kennedy, & Campis, 2021; Murray et al., 2023).

A key part of error management is understanding the difference between human error, risky behavior, and reckless conduct (Murray et al., 2023). Human error is unintentional, like Emily's medication omission due to unclear workflow processes, workload issues, or short staffing. Risky behavior involves taking shortcuts or ignoring procedures, which could stem from poor workplace design or high-pressure demands. In nursing, one of the most common examples of risky behavior involves "workarounds." Reckless conduct, however, is a deliberate disregard for safety protocols. Leaders must differentiate these categories to ensure responses are fair, proportional, and focused on learning rather than punishment. Upholders—leaders who are socially and organizationally aware—have the ability to recognize these nuances, using data, observation, and team insights to determine whether an error points to an individual's lapse or a larger system issue.

When we think about Just Culture, we can't forget to talk about events that never reach the patient. *Near misses* are hidden opportunities in healthcare—moments where an error almost happened but was caught in time. In a Just Culture, near misses are just as valuable as actual errors because they highlight system vulnerabilities before harm occurs. Take Emily, the ICU nurse who initially hesitated to report her medication mistake. If her hospital embraced Just Culture, near misses would be actively encouraged for reporting, allowing leadership to identify workflow inefficiencies and prevent future errors. Research shows that organizations with strong near-miss reporting systems experience fewer sentinel events, reinforcing that early detection leads to safer patient care (Murray et al., 2023). When healthcare teams view near misses as learning moments rather than close calls, they shift from reactive problem-solving to proactive safety improvements—and that's how real change happens. Refer to Figure 12 for an illustration of the causes and ways to handle each level of behavior.

The key takeaway? Accountability should focus on learning and prevention, not punishment (Lesandrini & Leclerc, 2024). When leaders embrace just culture and uphold psychological safety, healthcare workers become more engaged, transparent, and proactive about improving patient care. A socially and organizationally aware leader understands that errors aren't just the responsibility of one person—they reflect broader workplace challenges. By prioritizing systemic improvement over blame,

FIGURE 12

Human-centered leaders recognize the different levels of behavior of a just culture and aim to develop a culture of trust, excellence, and caring. Their actions are grounded in self-awareness, a learning mindset, psychological safety, and being socially and organizationally aware.

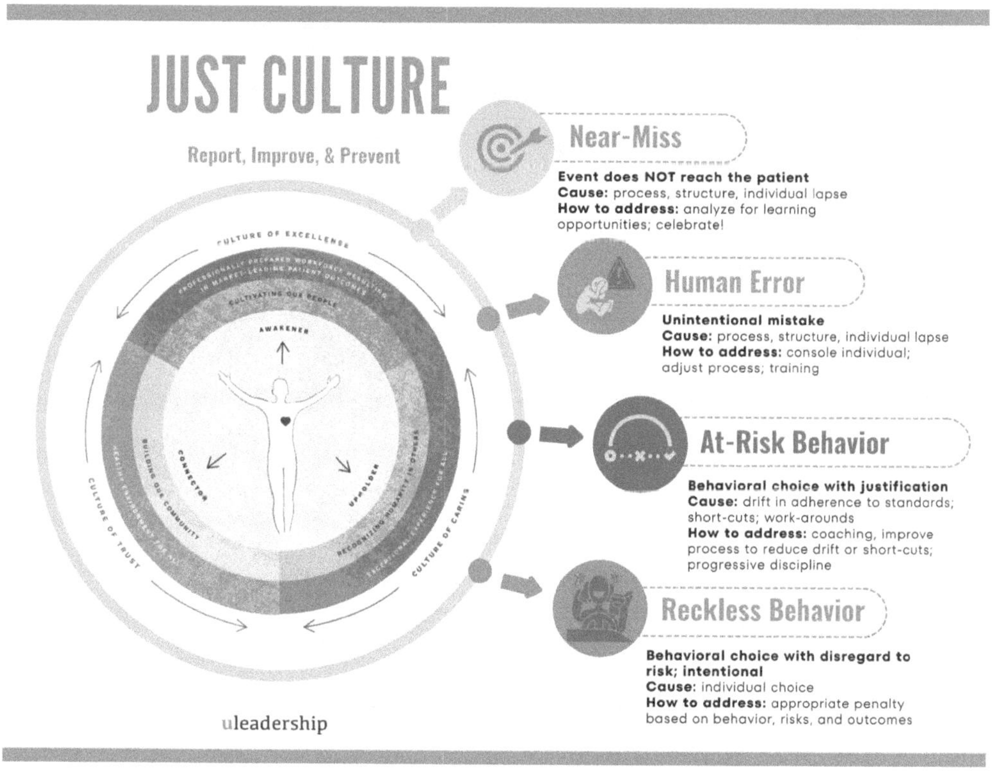

organizations foster a resilient, adaptive, and high-performing healthcare culture where staff feel safe to speak up, learn, and contribute to excellence.

Leadership Strategies to Embed Just Culture

Just culture doesn't just happen—it's built intentionally by leaders who model the way, set expectations, and create an environment where learning replaces fear. Take Emily, the ICU nurse who hesitated to report a medication omission because of a punitive culture. In an HCL framework, an authentic communicator (Connector) would have ensured clear expectations for error reporting, reinforcing that mistakes aren't career-ending—they're learning opportunities. Leaders who communicate transparently empower teams to speak up without hesitation, eliminating the silence that can lead to repeated errors (Adams, 2022; Välimäki et al., 2024).

But communication alone isn't enough. Leaders must model vulnerability and transparency themselves. A self-aware leader understands that errors are inevitable and responds with emotional intelligence rather than punitive action (Self and Upholder). Instead of viewing mistakes as personal failures, these leaders own their own missteps, showing staff that growth comes from reflection, not fear. According to van Baarle and colleagues (2022), when leaders can model how to synchronize emotions, perspectives, and facts, their teams will feel safe to do the same. Imagine if Emily's leadership had approached errors with honest dialogue instead of intimidation—she would have felt safe to report, leading to systemwide improvements rather than personal stress (Murray et al., 2023).

A culture of trust and excellence is the backbone of Just Culture, and leaders must build it through consistent accountability. An Awakener—who acts as both an architect and a coach—helps organizations move beyond top-down blame structures, shifting toward collaborative problem-solving. In Emily's case, structured peer reviews could have replaced punitive incident reports, allowing her team to collectively assess system flaws, rather than pointing fingers at individuals. Peer-driven assessments not only improve patient safety but also empower staff, reinforcing the idea that responsibility is shared, and solutions must be built together.

Ultimately, just culture is a leadership responsibility and one that demands intentional effort (Lesandrini & Leclerc, 2024; Kennedy, Leclerc, & Campis, 2021). Leaders must embody the behaviors they want to see, ensuring staff feel respected, supported, and encouraged to learn from mistakes rather than hide them. Whether through clear expectations (Connector), vulnerability and self-awareness (Self), emotional awareness (Upholder), or coaching-based leadership (Awakener), human-centered leaders set the tone for a psychologically safe workplace. And that safety doesn't just protect staff—it improves patient outcomes, transforming healthcare environments into spaces where learning thrives, and excellence is sustained.

Measuring Success in Implementing Just Culture

Just culture isn't just a philosophy—it's measurable. Healthcare organizations that implement just culture see tangible improvements in patient safety, staff engagement, and overall workplace well-being. One of the most critical metrics is increased reporting rates of errors and near misses. When staff feel psychologically safe, they are more likely to report mistakes, allowing leadership to identify patterns, address system flaws, and prevent future harm. A recent study using the Just Culture Assessment Tool found that a hospital with a strong just culture framework saw an increase in nurses' intention to voluntarily report errors (Paradiso & Sweeney, 2019). This shift is crucial because underreporting is one of the biggest barriers to improving patient safety—when errors go unreported, they repeat rather than resolve.

Let's revisit Emily, the ICU nurse who was hesitant to report her mistake due to fear of punishment. In a hospital that embraced Just Culture, Emily's experience would have been entirely different. Instead of fearing retaliation, she would have felt encouraged to report the issue, knowing that leadership would focus on systemwide improvements rather than individual blame. Over three years of just culture implementation, her hospital saw a 25% increase in employee retention, as staff felt more supported and engaged. Improved morale is another key metric—when healthcare professionals trust their leadership and feel safe to speak up, they are more engaged, collaborative, and committed to patient care.

Another powerful metric is the reduction in sentinel events and preventable harm. Hospitals that prioritize just culture see fewer catastrophic errors, as early reporting and systemwide learning help catch risks before they escalate. Research shows that organizations with strong just culture principles experience a decrease in preventable harm incidents, reinforcing that learning-driven accountability leads to safer patient outcomes (Adams, 2022; Kim & Yu, 2021; van Baarle et al., 2022). In Emily's hospital, structured peer reviews replaced punitive incident reports, allowing teams to collectively assess system flaws and refine workflows. This approach not only improved patient safety but also strengthened team collaboration, ensuring that errors became opportunities for growth rather than sources of fear.

The key takeaway? Just culture is measurable, and its impact is undeniable. Increased error reporting improves team morale and reduces sentinel events, proving that shifting from blame to learning transforms healthcare environments. Leaders who commit to just culture don't just improve workplace culture—they save lives. By embedding trust, transparency, and systemwide accountability, organizations create resilient, adaptive teams that thrive rather than just survive.

Embedding Just Culture for Long-Term Psychological Safety

Just culture isn't just a nice idea, it's a commitment to psychological safety that transforms how healthcare teams communicate, learn, and grow. Leaders who embrace HCL-HC—whether as Awakeners, Connectors, Upholders, or Self-led role models—create environments where trust replaces fear and accountability fosters improvement rather than punishment. Think of the hospital and leaders who rewrote the narrative in Emily's hospital, shifting the culture from blame to shared responsibility. Over time, error reporting increased, staff engagement soared, and patient safety improved. That transformation isn't just inspiring, it's possible anywhere with the right leadership approach. The call to action is simple: Start today. Set clear expectations, model vulnerability, build trust, and empower collaborative problem-solving. Healthcare leaders who embed just culture into their organizations don't just protect their teams—they build the future of safer, more compassionate care.

Discussion Questions for Groups

1. As a leadership team, what steps can you collectively take to foster a just culture where staff feel safe to report errors without fear? Consider how your organization currently handles mistakes and discuss specific strategies for shifting from punitive responses to learning-based accountability. How can you ensure psychological safety is embedded in leadership practices and daily operations?
2. HCL-HC's Connector focuses on building a culture of trust through authentic communication. How can nurse and healthcare leaders work together to strengthen team trust and transparency, ensuring that just culture principles are fully integrated into workplace policies and interactions? Explore how leaders at all levels can model vulnerability, encourage open dialogue, and create systems that reinforce shared responsibility over individual blame.

Reflection Questions for Individuals

1. Think about a time when you hesitated to report an error or concern in your workplace. What emotions influenced your decision, and how might a strong just culture have changed your response? Consider how trust, transparency, and leadership support could have created a different outcome.

    ____

    ____

    ____

    ____

    ____

2. How do you currently demonstrate HCL in fostering psychological safety within your team? What intentional actions can you take to strengthen trust, encourage open dialogue, and promote systemwide learning over individual blame? Reflect on how your leadership approach shapes team culture and error management practices.

    ____

    ____

    ____

    ____

    ____

References

Adams, D. E. (2022). Leadership for reducing medical errors via organizational culture: A literature review. *Measuring Business Excellence, 26*(2), 143–162. doi: 10.1108/MBE-06-2021-0079

American Nurses Association. (2024). *Fidelity in nursing: Ethical principles and professional commitment.* ANA. Retrieved from https://www.nursingworld.org

Elmi, A. H., Hassan, R. A., Abdi, A. O., Yusuf, F. Y., Ibrahim, K. H., & Abdi, A. A. (2025). Awareness of reporting practices and barriers to incident reporting among nurses in Mogadishu, Somalia. *BMC Nursing, 24*, Article 1134. doi: 10.1186/s12912-025-03799-y

Kennedy, K., Leclerc, L., & Campis, S. (2021). *Human-Centered Leadership in Healthcare: Evolution of a Revolution*. Morgan James Publishing.

Kim, B. B., & Yu, S. (2021). Effects of just culture and empowerment on patient safety activities of hospital nurses. *Healthcare (Basel, Switzerland), 9*(10), 1324. doi: 10.3390/healthcare9101324

Lansing, A. E., Romero, N. J., Siantz, E., Silva, V., Center, K., Casteel, D., & Gilmer, T. (2023). Building trust: Leadership reflections on community empowerment and engagement in a large urban initiative. *BMC Public Health, 23*(1), 1252. doi: 10.1186/s12889-023-15860-z

Lesandrini, J. & Leclerc, L. (2024). Fostering excellence in healthcare: The imperative for ethical leadership training in nurse leaders. *Nurse Leader, 22*(3), 273-277.

Murray, J. S., Clifford, J., Larson, S., Lee, J. K., & Sculli, G. L. (2023). Implementing just culture to improve patient safety. *Military Medicine, 188*(7–8), 1596–1599. doi: 10.1093/milmed/usac115

Paradiso, L., & Sweeney, N. (2019) Just culture: It's more than policy. *Nursing Management, 50*(6), 38–45. doi: 10.1097/01.NUMA.0000558482.07815.ae

Välimäki, M., Hu, S., Lantta, T., Hipp, K., Varpula, J., Chen, J., Liu, G., Tang, Y., Chen, W., & Li, X. (2024). The impact of evidence-based nursing leadership in healthcare settings: A mixed methods systematic review. *BMC Nursing, 23*, Article 452. doi: 10.1186/s12912-024-02096-4

van Baarle, E., Hartman, L., Rooijakkers, S., Wallenburg, I., Weenink, J.-W., Bal, R., & Widdershoven, G. (2022). Fostering a just culture in healthcare organizations: Experiences in practice. *BMC Health Services Research, 22*(1), 1035. doi: 10.1186/s12913-022-08418-z

Recommended Reading

Eng, D. M., & Schweikart, S. J. (2020). Why accountability sharing healthcare organizational cultures means patients are probably safer. *AMA Journal of Ethics, 22*(9), 779–783.

Institute for Safe Medication Practices. (2022). *Criminalization of human error and a guilty verdict: A travesty of justice that threatens patient safety*. Retrieved from https://www.ismp.org/resources/criminalization-human-error-and-guilty-verdict-travesty-justice-threatens-patient-safety

Institute of Medicine. (1999). *To err is human: Building a safer health system*. National Academies Press. doi: https://doi:10.17226/9728

Institute of Medicine. (2001). *Crossing the quality chasm.* National Academies Press. doi: https://doi:10.17226/10027

Leape, L. L. (1994). "Error in medicine." *Journal of the American Medical Association, 272,* 1851–1857.

Logroño, K. J., Al-Lenjawi, B. A., Singh, K., & Alomari, A. (2023). Assessment of nurse's perceived just culture: A cross-sectional study. *BMC Nursing, 22*(1), 348. doi: 10.1186/s12912-023-01478-4

National Council of State Boards of Nursing. (2012). *Just culture model for regulation.* Paper presented at the National Council of State Boards of Nursing Annual Meeting, Delegate Assembly. Retrieved from https://www.ncsbn.org/public-files/2012_Business_Book.pdf

Human-Centered Belonging

Human-Centered Belonging fosters collaboration and resilience by creating spaces where individuals feel valued and supported. *Teaming* empowers individuals to contribute their strengths toward shared goals, reinforcing a culture of inclusivity and collective success. *Dealing with joy interrupters* addresses challenges that threaten progress, using strategies rooted in resilience, mindfulness, and communal support to maintain positivity. Together with Human-Centered Leadership in Healthcare, these principles ensure that belonging is not just about inclusion but about flourishing in action, where individuals and teams thrive despite obstacles.

CHAPTER 18

Teaming

The Art of Collaboration

If you want to go fast, go alone. If you want to go far, go together.

—African proverb

In the complex, high-stakes environment of healthcare, successful outcomes are rarely the result of individual effort—it is built on the collective strength of a team. Teaming is the ability to work fluidly and adaptively with others, often in rapidly evolving situations. Unlike static teams with well-defined roles, effective teaming requires trust, communication, and an openness to learning from one another in real time.

Collaboration takes teamwork a step further, fostering an environment where diverse expertise converges to solve problems and drive innovation. It isn't just about working together, it's about engaging actively, sharing knowledge, and embracing different perspectives to find the best solutions.

At the foundation of both teaming and collaboration lies belonging. A culture of belonging ensures that every individual feels valued, empowered, and connected to a shared purpose. When people trust that their contributions matter and that their voices are heard, they engage more fully, take greater initiative, and commit to a higher standard of excellence. This sense of unity not only strengthens teams but also enhances patient care, allowing healthcare professionals to work seamlessly toward a common goal.

Flooded Floors, United Hearts: A Lesson in Teaming

One of the most unforgettable experiences I had as a nurse leader was during my time as the executive director of a burn unit. One afternoon, my nurse manager called me, her voice urgent, and said, “You need to get to the Burn ICU immediately . . . we’ve got a problem.”

When I arrived, the first thing that caught my eye was about a half inch of water covering the floor. Then, I heard it—the unmistakable sound of rushing water. I turned to my left and saw not just a drip, not even a steady stream, but a full-on torrent of water gushing from the ceiling. The ICU was flooded.

The Facilities Management team was already hard at work trying to stop the flow, but what unfolded over the next few hours was something I’ll never forget.

Within minutes, key leaders were at the scene: the vice president of the emergency department, the medical director of the burn unit, and the medical director of the hospital. Together, they quickly developed an action plan. Burn nurses stood vigilantly at every patient’s bedside, ensuring their safety. In what seemed like no time at all—truly, just minutes—the plan was set: move all 10 ICU patients to the Cardiac Cath postprocedure unit. This space wasn’t just large enough to accommodate everyone; it also had the necessary equipment, like EKG monitoring and oxygen systems, to support these critically ill patients.

And then, as if orchestrated by an invisible hand, people from every corner of the hospital jumped into action. Environmental services arrived to clean and prepare the new space. Respiratory therapists checked oxygen systems and prepped ventilators for transport. Transport teams appeared, ready to help move the patients. One by one, all 10 patients were safely relocated in what felt like record time.

But the teamwork didn’t stop there. When we arrived at the new unit, we were met by representatives from Central Supply, who had set up temporary supply carts tailored to the unique needs of burn patients. Pharmacy staff were on-site, establishing a temporary Pyxis system to ensure medications were readily accessible. IT teams were busy configuring computers to reflect the new unit setup. Even the unit secretary stepped in, making calls to patients’ families to explain what had happened and let them know where their loved ones had been moved.

Meanwhile, the burn unit nursing team held an impromptu meeting to sort out workflow adjustments, isolation precautions, and wound care logistics. Within a matter of a few hours, patients had been relocated, safe spaces equipped to meet their needs, supplies, and medications organized, and new workflows planned. It was a breathtaking example of teamwork, collaboration, and fortitude in action.

That day, I witnessed the most extraordinary example of "teaming" I've ever been a part of. The sense of accomplishment and belonging was overwhelming.

A huge shoutout to my Grady family—you showed me the true meaning of teamwork and belonging, and I'll carry that lesson with me always!

From Waterlogged to Wonder: The Power of Collaboration and Belonging

In the midst of chaos and confusion, like the burn unit flood, it's more than just teamwork at play—it's a moment that reflects a deeper sense of belonging. Each professional who rushes to the bedside isn't simply fulfilling their role; they're contributing to something greater, knowing that their skills, knowledge, and efforts matter, from environmental services to respiratory therapy to IT and Central Supply. There's an unspoken understanding among them: They are part of a collective, a team that relies on and supports each other. This connection fuels their ability to act swiftly and effectively, even under pressure. While teamwork is essential for executing tasks efficiently, collaboration thrives in environments that prioritize idea generation and problem-solving. Collaboration focuses on the process of working together, often with a higher degree of creativity and flexibility. It's about pooling ideas, sharing knowledge, and combining strengths to solve problems or innovate. Collaboration encourages active engagement, open communication, and collective decision-making.

Belonging is the foundation of collaboration. It's the feeling that every member of the team has a place, that their contributions are valued, and that they're united by a shared purpose. In healthcare, fostering a culture of belonging means creating an environment where every voice is heard, every role is respected, and every person feels they're an integral part of the mission.

When individuals feel they belong, they're more engaged and willing to collaborate, trusting that their unique perspectives and talents are appreciated. This culture of belonging doesn't just enhance teaming—it elevates the collective spirit, enabling professionals to work together seamlessly, just like the team in my experience. It's about more than saving lives or moving patients out of a flooded area into a safe area; it's about building a community where people support one another, knowing they're working toward something meaningful.

Where Belonging Fuels Collaboration

Dr. Amy Edmondson (2012), Harvard professor and author of *Teaming: How Organizations Learn, Innovate, and Compete in the Knowledge Economy*, states that the success or failure of complex organizations hinges on how effectively small groups within them operate. In healthcare, the delivery of exceptional patient care relies on teams and, increasingly, on flexible, adaptive collaborations that respond to evolving needs. With the rapid pace of advancements and the fluidity of modern healthcare systems, the emphasis has shifted from forming static, well-defined teams to mastering the art of leading effective teaming in dynamic, ever-changing environments. Think back to the collaboration and teaming that happened with the burn unit flood. Dr. Edmondson also identifies several barriers to successful teaming, both perceived and real. One of the biggest obstacles is fear of failure or blame, which can prevent individuals from speaking up, sharing ideas, or admitting mistakes. She emphasizes the importance of psychological safety, built on trust, where people feel safe to take risks and voice concerns without fear of punishment.

Another barrier is hierarchical structures and rigid roles, which can hinder collaboration and open communication. In environments where authority figures dominate decision-making, team members may hesitate to contribute, limiting innovation and problem-solving.

Additionally, competition over collaboration can hinder teaming. Many organizations foster a competitive mindset, which can make individuals reluctant to share knowledge or work together effectively.

And finally, Dr. Edmondson highlights the lack of shared goals and trust as a challenge. When team members do not have a clear, common purpose or do not trust one another, coordination and cooperation suffer. To overcome these barriers, she advocates for inclusive leadership, where leaders actively invite input, acknowledge their own vulnerability, and strive to create cultures of belonging.

A culture of collaboration and belonging thrives in an environment where teamwork, mutual respect, and shared goals shape every interaction. It's more than just working together—it's about building trust, fostering open communication, and embracing a shared sense of responsibility. In healthcare, this culture unites professionals from diverse disciplines, integrating their expertise to deliver comprehensive, patient-centered care.

At their core, human-centered leaders foster a culture where individuals feel empowered to share ideas, voice concerns, and acknowledge mistakes without fear of judgment. As Connectors, these leaders recognize that they don't need to have all the answers—they embrace collaboration, relying on the unique expertise and skills of their team to uncover solutions together. Their communication is clear, honest, and consistent, ensuring that everyone remains informed and aligned toward shared goals.

The Connector dimension exemplifies the essence of collaboration by supporting others, embracing change through ideas and innovation, and ensuring individuals are engaged in processes where their unique strengths can shine. Within this framework, every team member's contributions are not only acknowledged but also celebrated as integral to the group's success. These behaviors ultimately cultivate a culture of trust, where people feel valued and empowered to work together toward meaningful outcomes.

Patrick Lencioni (2002), in his classic work on teaming, *The Five Dysfunctions of a Team*, emphasizes that trust is the foundation of The Five Behaviors®, serving as the bedrock for meaningful collaboration and effective teamwork. Without trust, the collaboration vital for team success becomes elusive. True trust stems from vulnerability—a willingness to be authentic, open, and confident that colleagues will act with integrity and support one another.

By embodying the principles of a Connector, human-centered leaders cultivate collaborative teams through authentic communication, innovation, and mutual support. This approach creates a foundation for a Healthy Work Environment, as defined by the American Association of Critical Care Nurses (AACN, 2021), ensuring every team member thrives in a space built on trust and shared purpose (Figures 13 and 14; refer to Appendix H).

The Connector in Human-Centered Leadership plays a vital role in shaping functional teams and fostering a healthy work environment. As an **Authentic Communicator**, the Connector builds trust, creating the foundation for skilled communication that strengthens workplace culture. By serving as a **Collaborator**, the Connector navigates conflict effectively, ensuring teams master challenges together and cultivate true collaboration. This ability to guide productive discussions prevents tension from escalating and instead turns differences into opportunities for growth. Additionally, as an **Engineer** and **Edgewalker**, the Connector drives commitment within teams, helping them stay aligned with shared goals. This commitment fuels effective decision-making, reinforcing a culture where collaboration is not just encouraged but deeply embedded in the organization's fabric.

Beyond individual attributes, the Connector is a **Supporter** who embraces accountability, helping teams take ownership of their work while enhancing decision-making

FIGURE 13
Overcoming the Dysfunction of a Team as a Connector. Adapted from Lencioni (2002).

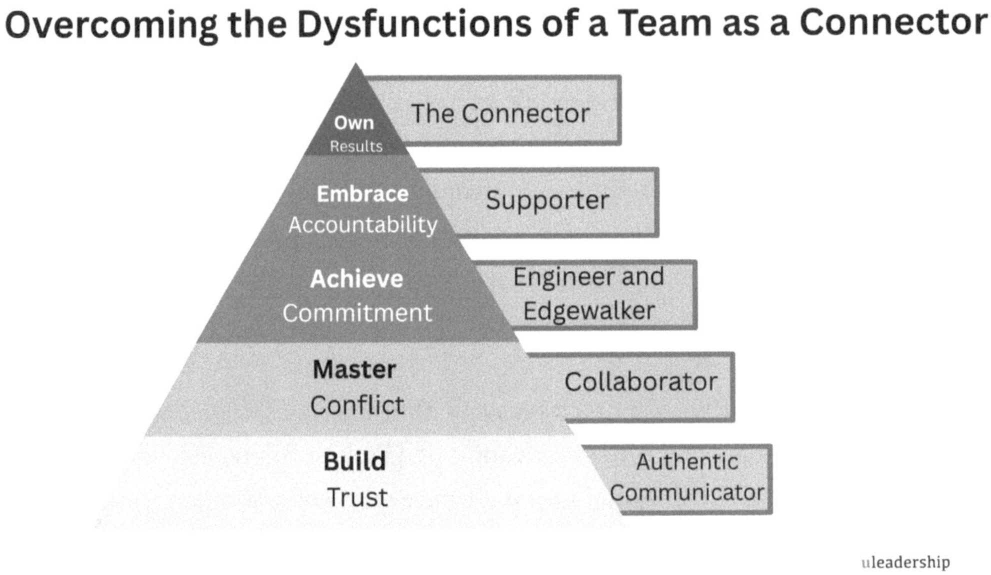

FIGURE 14
Connecting the Dots Between Human-Centered Leadership, Teaming, and a Healthy Work Environment. Adapted from Lencioni (2002).

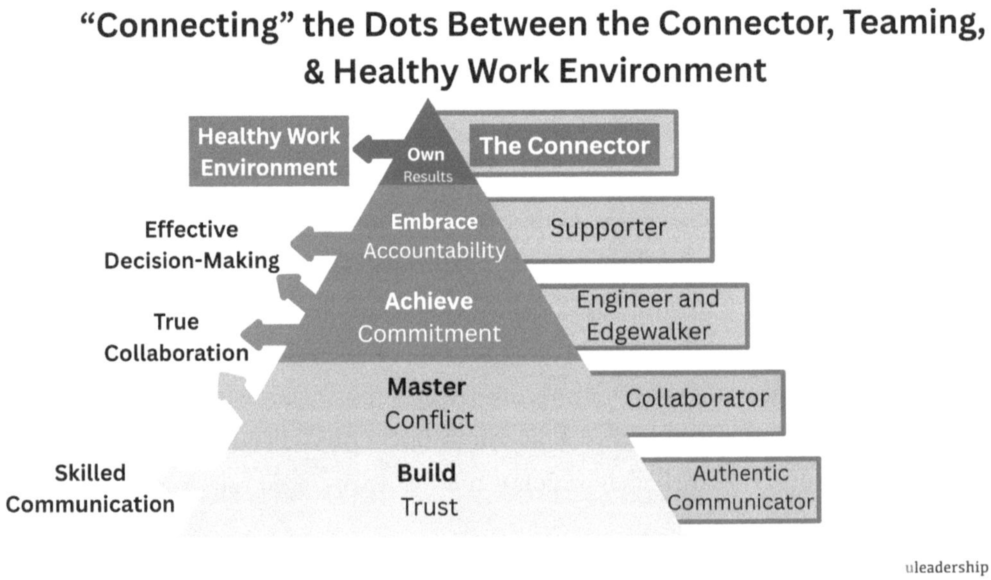

processes. When accountability is ingrained in a team's mindset, actions become more intentional, leading to improved patient care and workplace satisfaction. Ultimately, by embodying all these qualities, the Connector ensures that teams **own their results**, reinforcing a culture of responsibility, engagement, and purpose. This holistic approach transforms functional teams into thriving ecosystems, where psychological safety, trust, and collaboration drive a truly **healthy work environment**—one where individuals feel valued, heard, and empowered to contribute meaningfully.

By embracing collaboration, healthcare teams not only improve patient outcomes but also foster an inclusive environment of continuous learning, mutual respect, and innovation. This shared commitment creates a culture that extends beyond individual teams, elevating the entire healthcare community and inspiring better practices across disciplines.

Discussion Questions for Groups

1. How can healthcare teams cultivate vulnerability-based trust among members to ensure effective collaboration during high-pressure situations?
2. What strategies can leaders implement to create a sense of belonging for all team members, especially in diverse, multidisciplinary healthcare environments?
3. How does a mindset that embraces "I don't have to know it all" influence problem-solving and innovation in healthcare?
4. Reflecting on the burn unit flood, can you share an example where teaming and collaboration directly impacted patient outcomes, and what lessons can be applied to future practices?

Reflection Questions for Individuals

Think about a time when you were part of a team that worked exceptionally well together, especially in a healthcare setting or similar environment. Reflect on the following:

1. What aspects of trust and communication contributed to the team's success?
2. How did each member's unique contributions create a sense of belonging?
3. Were there moments of vulnerability or openness that strengthened the team dynamic?
4. How did collaboration influence the outcomes of the situation, particularly for those you were serving (e.g., patients)?

5. What lessons can you take from this experience to apply in future teamwork or leadership roles?

References

American Association of Critical Care Nurses. (2021). *Healthy work environments.* Retrieved from https://www.aacn.org

Edmondson, A. C. (2012). *Teaming: How organizations learn, innovate, and compete in the knowledge economy*. Jossey-Bass.

Lencioni, P. (2002). *The five dysfunctions of a team: A leadership fable.* Jossey-Bass.

Recommended Reading

Edmondson, A. C. (2018). *The fearless organization: Creating psychological safety in the workplace for learning, innovation, and growth.* John Wiley & Sons.

Edmondson, A. C. (2023). *Right kind of wrong: The science of failing well.* Atria Books.

Lencioni, P. M. (2016). *The ideal team player: How to recognize and cultivate the three essential virtues.* John Wiley & Sons.

CHAPTER 19

Dealing with Joy Interrupters

Flourishing in Action

Joy is much bigger than happiness. While happiness is often seen as being dependent on external circumstances, joy is not.

—Desmond Tutu, South African bishop, theologian, and human rights activist

You might love the concept of Human-Centered Leadership (HCL), but reality reminds us that not everyone leads this way. In fact, many leaders cling to traditional, transactional, or even toxic approaches. These approaches leave some team members feeling isolated and excluded. And let's be honest, healthcare has its fair share of staffing shortages, incivility, workplace frustrations, misaligned policies, and team dynamics that threaten to drain your joy. The American Nurses Association (ANA, 2023) has launched the Nurse Well-Being: Building Peer and Leadership Support Program, which provides evidence-based tools to help nurses recover from stress reactions, manage burnout, and foster resilience. This initiative recognizes that nurses face extraordinary stress, and it offers peer support, leadership training, and real-time resources to help nurses prioritize their well-being while continuing to provide high-quality care. Similarly, the American Association of Colleges of Nursing (2023) has issued a call to action for academic nurse leaders to promote well-being, resilience, and suicide prevention in nursing education and practice. Their initiative encourages building wellness cultures, offering mental health screenings, and implementing evidence-based interventions to support a healthy working and learning environment.

So, why all of the focus on well-being and joy? Let's address the elephant in the room. What happens when your joy is interrupted—not by circumstances, but by people? How do you stay true to your HCL approach when surrounded by individuals who see leadership differently? It's a real struggle. You might ask yourself, "What do I do when someone disrupts my joy?" While there's no one-size-fits-all answer, there are tangible, evidence-based strategies to help you maintain joy without losing your leadership identity. At the heart of this approach is self-awareness—choosing how to respond rather than reacting instinctively. And sometimes, that starts with recognizing how different leadership cultures influence joy.

A Story of Uninterrupted Joy . . . for the Most Part

When I first stepped into a nursing leadership role, I was welcomed by an organization that—while not perfect—valued collaboration, voice, and innovation. My direct supervisor, Monica, embodied HCL at every level. She wasn't just interested in metrics—she genuinely cared about how nurses felt in their roles. That approach trickled down into our everyday work. Under her leadership, we launched initiatives designed to give nurses ownership of patient outcomes. We introduced a mentorship program connecting new nurses with experienced leaders, helping them navigate their careers while strengthening community trust. Monica encouraged us to question outdated norms, sparking changes that empowered our ICU team, improved patient care, and ultimately built a culture of shared leadership.

But even in this environment, joy interrupters emerged. One example? The resistance to patient-centered rounding in our medical–surgical unit. Our goal was to shift traditional nurse rounding from a rigid checklist to a relational, trust-building approach. Instead of routine check-ins, nurses were encouraged to engage meaningfully, ensuring that patients felt heard rather than just assessed. Some nurses loved it. Others? Not so much. The skeptics argued:

- *"Patients expect quick check-ins, not long conversations. It slows us down."*
- *"We don't have time for this—we're stretched thin as it is."*
- *"This isn't how we've ever done it. Why change something that works?"*

Monica didn't dismiss their concerns—she listened first. She provided evidence-based research showing that patient-centered communication improves outcomes. Then, she piloted the new rounding process gradually, allowing nurses to adapt without pressure. Within months, the skeptics saw the impact firsthand: Patients felt calmer, family members were more engaged, and nurses reported stronger relationships with their patients. Even the most resistant staff members admitted, "I never realized how much difference real conversation makes. I wouldn't go back."

Taking Action: How Do I Protect My Joy?

Patience: The Power of the Pause

In healthcare, few conflicts or leadership challenges are resolved instantly. Patience is a leadership skill that requires self-awareness and emotional intelligence, allowing leaders to pause, assess perspectives, and respond thoughtfully rather than react impulsively. According to Spanos, Smith, and Taylor (2024), effective healthcare leaders navigate complexity by fostering collaboration and building cultures of capacity. This means that when confronted with traditional, transactional, or toxic leadership behaviors, the human-centered leader chooses to redirect the conversation to a time when emotions are settled, ensuring a productive and professional dialogue.

Take Robert, an ICU director who championed open visitation. He knew that buy-in wouldn't happen overnight, so instead of forcing change, he patiently guided his team toward understanding the benefits. He didn't impose a rigid timeline—he invited nurses to explore the evidence and make their own informed decisions.

Kindness: A Leadership Superpower

You've probably seen the phrase "Choose Kind" on T-shirts and billboards, but in healthcare leadership, kindness is more than a slogan—it's a strategy. Research by Dyar, Chen, and Parker (2024) highlights that kindness in leadership fosters psychological safety, improves team dynamics, and enhances patient care. When faced with resistance or conflict, responding with kindness, confidence, and evidence-based reasoning can de-escalate tension and create space for meaningful dialogue.

Patterson et al. (2012) outlined six tactics for navigating crucial conversations with kindness and heart as starting points. Although these were developed a while back, these strategies stand the test of time and remain relevant today.

1. **Start with the Heart**—Align your motives with the shared goal of *quality patient care.*
2. **Learn to Look**—Recognize emotional escalation and *redirect the conversation* when needed.
3. **Make It Safe**—Reinforce *common ground and shared purpose* to maintain a respectful dialogue.
4. **Master Your Story**—Separate *personal assumptions from reality* to avoid unnecessary conflict.
5. **State Your Path and Explore Others'**—Focus on *facts and evidence*, inviting others to do the same.
6. **Move to Action**—Ensure that every conversation leads to *clear next steps and accountability.*

Kindness isn't about passivity—it's about leading with integrity and fostering environments where people feel valued. Greco, Sanchez, and Patel (2025) reinforce that kindness-based leadership interventions improve workplace culture and reduce burnout.

Be Intentional: Leading with Purpose

Intentional leadership is about making conscious choices—whether it's setting the tone for a meeting, responding to a difficult colleague, or shaping workplace culture. According to Pattali, Green, and Martinez (2024), leaders who intentionally cultivate trust and empowerment reduce turnover and improve nurse engagement.

Human-centered leaders use intention as a proactive tool to navigate challenges. For example, when working with a micromanaging executive director, setting a daily intention—such as "Pause, be present, and listen before responding"—can shift interactions from reactive to constructive. Over time, these intentional practices become second nature, reinforcing calm, confident leadership. Journaling and reflection can further strengthen intentional leadership, helping leaders track progress, refine strategies, and stay accountable to their values.

Do What's Right, Every Time: Ethical Leadership

At the core of HCL is a simple principle: Do what's right. Dr. Mishra, a revered chief medical officer, embodied this philosophy—whether advocating for patients, supporting staff, or navigating complex healthcare decisions. His approach aligns with Välimäki, Johnson, and Lee (2024), who emphasize that ethical and evidence-based leadership improves both clinical and organizational outcomes.

The ANA Code of Ethics (2024) reinforces this principle by emphasizing human flourishing and ethical decision-making as foundational to nursing practice. Provisions within the updated code stress that nurses must advocate for environments that promote well-being, dignity, and equitable care, ensuring that ethical choices are not just reactive but proactively embedded into leadership practices. Doing what's right extends beyond individual actions—it's about creating systems where ethical behavior is the norm, not the exception. Leaders like Dr. Mishra exemplify this by making decisions that prioritize patients, colleagues, and the broader healthcare community, aligning their leadership with both evidence-based outcomes and moral integrity. When nurses and healthcare professionals champion human flourishing, they transform workplaces into spaces where both staff and patients feel valued, supported, and empowered to thrive.

When faced with joy interrupters, human-centered leaders pause, speak calmly, and uphold ethical decision-making. Fidelity (the commitment to quality, compassionate care) is central to nursing leadership (ANA, 2024). Whether advocating for open visitation, equitable staffing, or patient-centered policies, leaders who consistently do what's right build trust, resilience, and lasting impact (refer to Figure 15).

Joy Interrupted, But Not Lost

Belonging is the heartbeat of joy in healthcare leadership. Fredrickson's (2009) 3-to-1 positivity ratio reminds us that cultivating three positive emotions for every negative experience creates a tipping point for joy flourishing. But joy isn't just about individual mindset, it's about leaders actively fostering an environment where every team member feels valued, heard, and safe to contribute. Human-centered leaders can strengthen belonging by embedding patience, kindness, intentionality, and ethical decision-making into daily interactions. A leader's words, actions, and willingness to create space for others determine whether teams thrive or merely survive.

FIGURE 15
Protecting your joy is a priority for sustainable leadership. Human-centered leaders harness the power of Patience, Kindness, Intention, and Ethical Leadership to deal with the "joy interrupters" in their workplace.

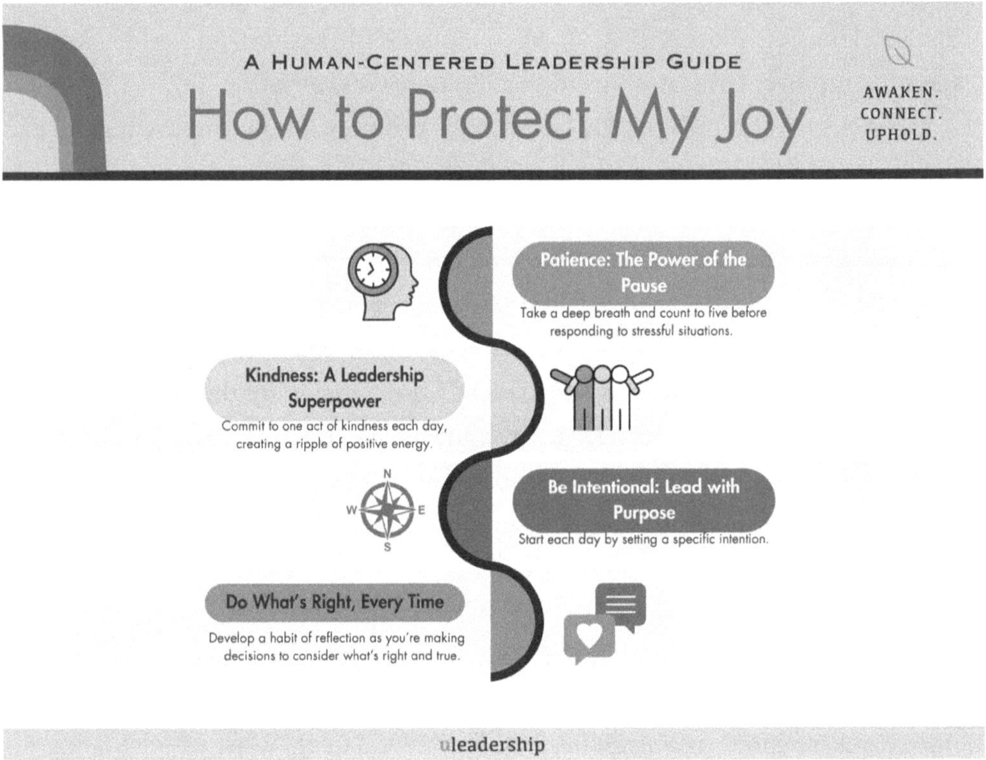

When workplace stress, toxic leadership, or difficult conversations arise, the presence or absence of belonging shapes how teams respond. Leaders who prioritize psychological safety and create trust-filled environments not only counteract negativity but also build cultures of inclusion where individuals feel connected rather than isolated. Belonging fosters engagement, innovation, and stronger relationships, ensuring staff and patients alike flourish in an environment of mutual support. Research shows that teams with high psychological safety and a strong sense of belonging report fewer errors, experience lower burnout rates, and demonstrate greater commitment to shared goals (Murray et al., 2023).

Here's the key takeaway: Joy and belonging are inseparable in healthcare leadership. Even when surrounded by skepticism or rigid hierarchies, human-centered leaders can shape environments where inclusion fuels resilience. The strongest teams aren't perfect—they're adaptive, courageous, and willing to rethink outdated ways of working. Protecting joy isn't about avoiding challenges, it's about navigating them in a way that reinforces connection, accountability, and shared purpose.

By embracing intentional positivity, fostering trust, and leading with empathy, human-centered leaders create workplaces where people don't just show up—they belong. And when belonging is woven into leadership choices, joy is no longer fleeting—it becomes a lasting force for transformation, well-being, and excellence in healthcare.

Discussion Questions for Groups

1. How can leaders cultivate patience and kindness in high-stress healthcare environments, especially when faced with resistance or negativity? Reflect on a time when patience and kindness helped resolve a leadership challenge or interpersonal conflict. What strategies can leaders implement to ensure these qualities remain central to their leadership approach, even in moments of frustration or urgency?
2. In what ways can intentionality and ethical decision-making shape a workplace culture that protects joy and supports human flourishing? Discuss real-world examples of how leaders have intentionally designed policies, conversations, or workflows that prioritize staff well-being and ethical integrity. How can leaders ensure joy isn't an afterthought, but rather an embedded part of organizational decision-making?

Reflection Questions for Individuals

1. Think about a time when someone or something interrupted your joy in the workplace. How did you respond, and in hindsight, what could you have done differently using patience and intentionality? Consider how taking a moment to pause, adjusting your perspective, or setting clear intentions might have shaped the outcome more positively.

____

____

____

____

____

2. How do you currently integrate kindness and ethical decision-making into your leadership or daily interactions? Reflect on a moment when you actively chose to lead with kindness and do what's right despite challenges. What impact did that choice have on yourself, your colleagues, or your work environment?

____

____

____

____

____

References

American Association of Colleges of Nursing. (2023). *Well-being & resilience initiative: Supporting mental health in nursing education and practice.* AACN. Retrieved from https://www.aacnnursing.org/our-initiatives/well-being-resilience

American Nurses Association. (2023). *Nurse well-being: Building peer and leadership support program.* ANA. Retrieved from https://www.nursingworld.org/foundation/programs/nurse-wellbeing

American Nurses Association. (2024). *Fidelity in nursing: Ethical principles and professional commitment.* ANA. Retrieved from https://www.nursingworld.org

Dyar, R., Chen, L., & Parker, A. (2024). Kindness in healthcare leadership and management: An evaluation and analysis of the concept. *BMJ Leader, 9*(1), 77–93. doi: 10.1136/leader-2023-000742

Fredrickson, B. L. (2009). *Positivity: Groundbreaking research reveals how to embrace the hidden strength of positive emotions, overcome negativity, and thrive.* Crown Publishing.

Greco, P., Sanchez, F., & Patel, N. (2025). What's the role of kindness in the healthcare context? A scoping review. *BMC Health Services Research, 29*(4), 102–117. doi: 10.1186/s12913-025-12328-1

Pattali, V., Green, T., & Martinez, S. (2024). Effect of leadership styles on turnover intention among staff nurses in private hospitals. *BMC Health Services Research, 28*(2), 88–103. doi: 10.1186/s12913-024-10674-0

Spanos, A., Smith, J., & Taylor, L. (2024). Healthcare leaders navigating complexity: A scoping review of key trends in future roles and competencies. *BMC Medical Education, 24*(3), 45–60. doi: 10.1186/s12909-024-05689-4

Välimäki, M., Johnson, R., & Lee, K. (2024). The impact of evidence-based nursing leadership in healthcare settings: A mixed methods systematic review. *BMC Nursing, 23*(1), 12–29. doi: 10.1186/s12912-024-02096-4

Recommended Reading

Institute for Healthcare Improvement. (2024). *IHI framework for improving joy in work.* Retrieved from https://www.ihi.org/resources/white-papers/ihi-framework-improving-joy-work

Leape, L. (2013). *Through the eyes of the workforce: Creating joy, meaning, and safer health care.* Institute for Healthcare Improvement. Retrieved from https://www.ihi.org/resources/publications/through-eyes-workforce-creating-joy-meaning-and-safer-health-care

Wheat, S. (2024, October 3). *Reclaiming joy in health care: Taking control amidst systemic challenges.* KevinMD. Retrieved from https://www.kevinmd.com/2024/10/reclaiming-joy-in-health-care-taking-control-amidst-systemic-challenges.html

PART V

The Journey Continues

The evolution of Human-Centered Leadership in Healthcare isn't just an abstract movement—it's an active, ongoing revolution, shaped by leaders who prioritize well-being for Self and then face outward to Awaken, Connect, and Uphold others. Every healthcare professional has a role in driving this change by championing relational leadership and ensuring systemic improvements that prioritize human dignity over rigid hierarchies. This transformation starts with small, intentional actions—encouraging open dialogue, modeling vulnerability, and empowering teams to challenge outdated norms. The call to action is clear: lead boldly, communicate authentically, and build workplaces where people don't just work, they belong and flourish. In this shared effort, we don't just observe change, we become the architects of a healthcare future built on trust, resilience, and compassion.

CHAPTER 20

The Tipping Point Is Just Ahead . . .

The tipping point is that magic moment when an idea, trend, or social behavior crosses a threshold, tips, and spreads like wildfire.

—Malcolm Gladwell, Canadian journalist and acclaimed writer

We're no longer just imagining what Human-Centered Leadership in Healthcare (HCL-HC) could look like, we're standing at the tipping point, where the movement is unfolding in real time. The shift from hierarchical, transactional leadership to trust-driven, relational leadership isn't theoretical anymore, it's happening in hospitals, clinics, and healthcare systems that recognize that people, not processes, drive lasting change. Leaders who once focused solely on metrics and efficiency are now embracing belonging, psychological safety, and ethical accountability as essential pillars of healthcare excellence.

This tipping point isn't just about policies or strategies, it's about leaders making different choices every day (Gladwell, 2002, 2024). It's about redefining accountability as learning, shifting conversations from compliance to connection, and moving from fear-based management to environments where staff can thrive. The real revolution in Human-Centered Leadership (HCL) is found not in grand theories but in small, intentional actions—a leader modeling vulnerability, a team embracing peer-driven learning, and an organization committing to systemic improvement over punitive responses.

Healthcare teams are demanding change, not passively waiting for it. Nurses, physicians, and administrators alike are calling for leadership that honors the complexity of human experience, one that prioritizes trust and collaboration over rigid control structures. The era of fear-based leadership and disengagement is breaking down, replaced by an approach that centers on people, relationships, and collective resilience.

This is the moment to fully embrace HCL-HC, not as an ideal to strive for, but as the new standard for healthcare organizations. The tipping point has arrived, and those willing to lean into this transformation will be the ones who build a future where leadership is less about managing tasks and more about cultivating environments where both staff and patients truly flourish.

Be the Pebble in the Pond

Change in healthcare leadership doesn't always come in sweeping, dramatic shifts. It often begins with small, intentional actions that ripple outward, influencing the entire system. Imagine dropping a single pebble into a pond. At first, it's just a splash, but soon, waves begin expanding, reaching farther than expected. That's how HCL works—change starts from within (Self), then extends outward to Awaken, Connect, and Uphold the larger healthcare culture. The chaos and unpredictability of healthcare aren't barriers to change, they're catalysts. Every decision a leader makes, no matter how small, sets off a ripple effect, shaping the environment around them.

As a nurse leader, your daily choices influence far more than your immediate team. Think back to Emily, the ICU nurse who hesitated to report a medication mistake. A Self-led leader, one who models vulnerability and ethical reflection, might start by encouraging open conversations around errors. That leader's honesty ripples outward, Awakening teams to rethink punitive responses, Connecting staff by building trust, and ultimately Upholding systemic change that shifts how the organization views accountability. Over time, error reporting increases, fear decreases, and the workplace culture transforms. It's proof that leadership isn't just about authority, it's about small, intentional acts that create lasting impact.

Embracing chaos as the edge of change is where leadership growth happens. When faced with disruptions—staffing shortages, new policies, unforeseen challenges—leaders can either resist or adapt. Chaos is the space where, you, as a leader, get to choose how to react and adapt. You get the choice of resisting chaos and change or welcoming it with a mindful and authentic presence. As a human-centered leader, you choose the latter and pave a new way not just for the individual or the unit but for the entire system or organization. Consider a nurse manager implementing a hospital-wide hourly rounding mandate. Instead of forcing a rigid, one-size-fits-all model, they could pause, listen, and refine, advocating for small unit-based adjustments to ensure the policy supports patient care rather than disrupts workflows. That single decision—choosing collaboration over compliance—creates a ripple effect, improving both patient and nurse satisfaction and strengthening trust between staff and leadership.

Not every innovation requires a massive overhaul or a groundbreaking discovery. Often, the smallest shifts create the most profound impact. Human-centered leaders recognize that change doesn't start at the organizational level, it starts within individuals who choose to lead differently. Self-awareness drives intentional actions, Awakeners inspire reflection, Connectors build trust, and Upholders ensure stability. Drop the pebble. Be the pebble. Start the ripple. And watch as leadership choices, made with presence, empathy, and courage, expand far beyond the moment, creating lasting waves of transformation in healthcare.

> To learn more on how to be part of the HCL movement, please visit our website: www.uleadership.com. Also, consider testing the theory against journey to excellence metrics. We would love to partner with you in this revolution.

Momentum

Momentum doesn't begin with sweeping reforms. It starts with one small, intentional act that sparks something bigger. Think about the story of the starfish thrower, a simple yet powerful parable of change. A man walking along a beach sees thousands of stranded starfish, slowly drying out under the Sun. A child ahead of him is picking them up one by one and tossing them back into the ocean. The man tells the child, *"There are too many—there's no way you can save them all. You won't make a difference."* Without hesitation, the child picks up another starfish, throws it into the water, and says, "It made a difference to that one."

That's how movements begin. Not from grand gestures, but from someone, just one person, choosing to act. In healthcare leadership, HCL is gaining momentum not because systems suddenly transformed overnight, but because leaders are making small but meaningful choices that ripple outward. A nurse leader who models vulnerability (Self), an Awakener who inspires growth, a Connector who fosters trust, and an Upholder who nurtures belonging—each of these actions may seem small, but together, they build the foundation for a healthcare culture that prioritizes people over rigid structures.

We challenge you to be the starfish thrower, no matter how overwhelming change may seem. You don't have to overhaul your leadership style tomorrow—you can start by recognizing the humanity in yourself and in others. Advocate for psychological safety, engage in authentic conversations, and choose trust over fear in your interactions. Over time, these moments add up, shifting the tide in healthcare leadership from metrics-driven to human-centered.

Imagine if just one nurse in every hospital embraced this approach—then another, then another. With four million nurses in the United States alone, the ripple effect would be unstoppable. The world doesn't need a single hero. It needs many committed individuals making small but significant choices every day. And with those choices, HCL-HC moves from an idea into a revolution, one where healthcare professionals don't just work within systems, they shape them for the better.

Don't Let Anything or Anyone Stop You

You may have recognized yourself in the dimensions of the Awakener, the Connector, and the Upholder, perhaps even thinking, *"I already do most of this."* That's a powerful realization, but the real tipping point happens when leaders pause and ask: Am I neglecting myself in this process? We've seen firsthand what happens when healthcare leaders focus only on serving others—we "gave" until burnout set in, forgetting that sustainable leadership begins within. Without prioritizing our own well-being, reflection, and psychological safety, the ripples we create eventually weaken, leaving us exhausted instead of empowered.

HCL-HC is at a tipping point, not just an abstract idea but a movement that's shifting the foundation of healthcare. We've spent years imagining and bringing to life what a human-centered leader could look like, and now, change is happening in real time. It's tempting to believe transformation requires large-scale action, but in reality, every movement starts with a single ripple. Think of the pebble dropped into a pond—one small act creates waves that stretch far beyond what's immediately visible. That's how leadership works. Each choice, each conversation, and each moment of trust-building adds momentum, pushing healthcare closer to a future where people, not policies, drive excellence.

This is your moment to step into the ripple effect, to recognize that change isn't just happening, it's waiting for you to take part. The strongest teams, the most impactful leaders, and the most resilient organizations aren't perfect, they're adaptive, intentional, and committed to rethinking outdated ways of working. Healthcare leadership isn't just about meeting metrics, it's about cultivating environments where people thrive. And that begins with one small act—the pebble in the pond—that sets everything in motion.

Discussion Questions for Groups

1. Leadership is often viewed as large-scale transformation, but real change begins with small, intentional actions—the "pebble in the pond" effect. What small leadership choices have you made that created unexpected ripples within your team or organization? How can leaders amplify these moments to push healthcare toward the tipping point of HCL-HC?
2. Healthcare is at a tipping point—a moment where the shift from transactional leadership to trust-driven, HCL-HC is gaining momentum. As a leader, how can you actively contribute to this movement? What systemic barriers might slow progress, and how can teams collectively overcome them to sustain lasting change?

Reflection Questions for Individuals

What's one small leadership habit or mindset shift you can commit to today that might create a ripple effect in your workplace? How can you stay accountable for making this change and ensuring it contributes to the larger movement of HCL-HC?

References

Gladwell, M. (2002). *The tipping point: How little things can make a big difference.* Back Bay Books.

Gladwell, M. (2024). *Revenge of the tipping point: Overstories, superspreaders, and the rise of social engineering.* Little, Brown.

Recommended Reading

Albert, N. M., Pappas, S., Porter-O'Grady, T., & Malloch, K. (2020). *Quantum leadership: Creating sustainable value in health care* (6th ed.). Jones & Bartlett Learning.

APPENDIX A

Publications on Human-Centered Leadership in Healthcare (2020 to 2024)

	Year	Reference
1	2024	Heier, C., Leclerc, L., Sanner-Stiehr, E., Busenhart, C., Park, S. H., & Nelson-Brantley, H. (2024). Improving nurse faculty job satisfaction: An action guide for academic nurse leaders. *Journal of Professional Nursing, 55*, 73–80.
2	2024	Leclerc, L., & Hoffman, C. (2024, July/August). An exemplar in honoring the shared human experience: Nurse honor guards. *Georgia Nursing, 84*(3), 5.
3	2024	Campis, S., Leclerc, L., & Kennedy, K. (2024). Inspiring and nurturing Human-Centered Leaders: The vital role of mentorship. *Journal of Continuing Education in Nursing, 5*, 276–278.
4	2024	Leclerc, L., D'Aquino, V., Lance, L., & Poole, V. (2024). Blending science, technology, and humanity: The dynamic role of radiology nursing. *Journal of Radiology Nursing, 43*(4), 235 239.
5	2024	Sipe, M. H. & Kennedy, K. (2024). Integrating human-centered approaches to align Doctor of Nursing Practice curriculum with real-world practice. *Nurse Leader*, *22*(3), 209–302.
6	2024	Lesandrini, J., & Leclerc, L. (2024). Fostering excellence in healthcare: The imperative for ethical leadership training in nurse leaders. *Nurse Leader, 22*(3), 273–277.
7	2024	Raso, R., Bailey, K. D., Fitzpatrick, J., Kennedy, K., & Leclerc, L. (2024). Bold inquiry into relational leadership. *Nursing Management, 55*(1), 7–8. doi: 10.1097/nmg .0000000000000085
8	2023	Kennedy, K. (2024). Leadership style matters. *American Nurse, 19*(3), 48–48. doi:10.51256/ anj032448
9	2023	Leclerc, L., Bailey, K. D., Fitzpatrick, J., Kennedy, K., & Raso, R. (2023). Getting schooled in relational leadership. *Journal of Nursing Education, 62*(11), 599–600. doi: 10.3928 /01484834-20231010-02

	Year	Reference
10	2023	Leclerc, L., & Pabico, C. (2023). A blueprint for well-being: Modeling the way through Human-Centered Leadership and Pathway to Excellence. *Nursing Management, 54*(4), 9–16. doi: 10.1097/01.NUMA.0000921892.27917.78
11	2023	Leclerc, L., Kennedy, K., & Campis, S. (2023). Cultural intelligence (CQ): Flex your CQ muscle through a human-centered leadership workout! *Nurse Leader, 21*(3), 362–365.
12	2023	Kennedy, K., Leclerc, L., & Campis S. (2023). Human-centered leadership. In J. J. Fitzpatrick & C. M. Alfes (Eds.), *Nurse leadership and management: Foundations for executive administration* (pp. 552–554). Springer Publishing.
13	2022	Kennedy, K., Leclerc, L., & Campis, S. (2022). The great realization: Nurses are in the driver's seat. *Nurse Leader, 20*(5), 480–484. doi: 10.1016/j.mnl.2022.05.011
14	2022	Leclerc, L., Strenge-McNabb, K., Thibodeaux, T., Campis, S., & Kennedy, K. (2022). Relational leadership: A contemporary and evidence-based approach to improve nursing work environments. *Nursing Management, 53*(7), 24–34. doi: 10.1097/01.NUMA.0000834580.84896.55
15	2022	Campis, S., Kennedy, K., & Leclerc, L. (2022, Sept/Oct). Human-centered leadership in action: Embracing healthy boundaries. *Georgia Nursing, 82*(4), 6.
16	2022	Campis, S., Kennedy, K., & Leclerc, L. (2022, July/August). Human-centered leadership in action: One turtle at a time. *Georgia Nursing, 83*(3), 9.
17	2021	Kennedy, K., Leclerc, L., & Campis, S. (2021a). *Human-centered leadership in healthcare: Evolution of a revolution*. Morgan James Publishing.
18	2021	Kennedy, K., Leclerc, L., & Campis, S. (2021b). *Shifts, the journal for nurses, by nurses*. Morgan James Publishing.
19	2021	Leclerc L., Kennedy K., & Campis S. (2021). Human-centered leadership in health care: A contemporary nursing leadership theory generated via constructivist grounded theory. *Journal of Nursing Management, 29*(2), 294–306. doi: 10.1111/jonm.13154
20	2020	Leclerc, L., Kennedy, K., & Campis, S. (2020). Human-centered leadership in health care: An idea that's time has come. *Nursing Administration Quarterly, 44*(2), 117–126.
21	2020	Kennedy, K., Campis, S., & Leclerc, L. (2020). Human-centered leadership: Creating change from the inside out. *Nurse Leader, 18*(3), 227–231. doi: 10.1016/j.mnl.2020.03.009

APPENDIX B

Global Citations—Human-Centered Leadership in Healthcare

	Year	Publication	Work Cited	Country—
1	2021	Fennell, K. (2021). Conceptualisations of leadership and relevance to health and human service workforce development: A scoping review. *Journal of Multidisciplinary Healthcare, 14*, 3035–3051.	Leclerc, Kennedy, & Campis (2020)	**Australia** -University of Tasmania
2	2022	Backes, D. S., Zinhani, M. C., Erdmann, A. L., Backes, M. T., Büscher, A., & Marchiori, M. R. (2022). Nursing care as a systemic and entrepreneurial phenomenon. *Journal of the School of Nursing—University of São Paulo, 56*, e20220249.	Leclerc, Kennedy, & Campis (2021)	**Brazil** -Universidade Franciscana -Universidade Federal de Santa Catarina **Germany** -Hochschule Osnabrück
3	2022	Hawksworth, L. T., Raja, S., Drake, J., Davis, T., O'Brien, A.-M., & Brady, J. M. (2022). Exploring nurses' perceptions of the barriers and facilitators that influence acceptance and use of remote visual monitoring technology. *Journal of Nursing Management, 30*(7), 1–15.	Leclerc, Kennedy, & Campis (2021)	**United States** -George Mason University
4	2022	Polanco-Diges, L., Saura, J. R., & Pinto, P. (2022). Setting the relationship between human-centered approaches and users' digital well-being: A review. *Journal of Tourism, Sustainability, and Well-Being, 10*(3), 148–171.	Kennedy, Campis, & Leclerc (2020)	**Spain** -Rey Juan Carlos University **Portugal** -University of Algarve

	Year	Publication	Work Cited	Country—
5	2022	Purcell, J. W., Rodriguez, D. X., & Ring, K. A. (2022). The Covid Shift: Working women's punctuated equilibrium. *Leadership & Organization Development Journal, 43*(8), 1217–1233.	Leclerc, Kennedy, & Campis, (2020)	**United States** -Kennesaw State University
6	2022	Singh, A., Mane, M., Mohanty, M. D., & Sharma, A. K. (2022). Exploring the mediating role of quality factors between healthcare leadership and patient satisfaction. *Health Leadership and Quality of Life, 1,* 118. doi: 10.56294/hl2022118	Leclerc, Kennedy, & Campis (2021)	**India** -Noida International University
7	2022	Stievano, A., Mynttinen, M., Rocco, G., & Kangasniemi, M. (2022). Public health nurses' professional dignity: An interview study in Finland. *Nursing Ethics, 29*(6), 1503–1517.	Leclerc, Kennedy, & Campis (2021)	**Italy** -Alessandro Scievano Dept. of Nursing
8	2022	Zhang, F., Peng, X., Huang, L., Liu, Y., Xu, J., He, J., Guan, C., Chang, H., & Chen, Y. (2022). A caring leadership model in nursing: A grounded theory approach. *Journal of Nursing Management, 30*(4), 981–992. doi: 10.1111/jonm.13600	Leclerc, Kennedy, & Campis (2021)	**China** -Union Hospital; Tongji Medical College -School of Nursing Tongji Medical College -Huazhong University of Science and Technology
9	2023	Blaustein, M., & Garelli, F. M. (2023). What about health education? Hegemony, paradigms in tension and alternatives. *Frontiers in Medicine, 10,* 1289865. doi: 10.3389/fmed.2023.1289865	Leclerc, Kennedy, & Campis (2021)	**Argentina** -Universidad de Buenos Aires
10	2023	Featherbe, R. (2023). Restorative clinical supervision: A chance for change but are we ready? *British Journal of Nursing, 32*(11), 514–520	Leclerc, Kennedy, & Campis (2021)	**England** -Torbay and South Devon NHS Foundation Trust
11	2023	Godfrey, N., & Joseph, M. L. (2023). Rebuilding professional identity: The time is now. *Nurse Leader, 21*(2), 179–182.	Kennedy, Leclerc, & Campis (2022)	**United States** -University of Kansas
12	2023	Grubaugh, M. L., Africa, L., & Loresto, F. L. (2023). Exploring the relationship between psychological capital and turnover among new nurses. *Nurse Leader, 21*(3), 409–414.	Leclerc, Kennedy, & Campis (2021)	**United States** -University of Colorado
13	2023	Jubinville, M., Tchouaket, E. N., & Longpré, C. (2023). Scoping review protocol examining charge nurse skills: Requirement for the development of training. *BMJ Open, 13,* e067307. doi:10.1136/bmjopen-2022-067307	Kennedy, Leclerc, & Campis (2021)	**Canada** - Université du Québec

	Year	Publication	Work Cited	Country—
14	2023	Lee, M. C. C., Kee, Y. J., Lau, S. S. Y., & Jan, G. (2023). Investigating aspects of paternalistic leadership within the job demands-resources model. *Journal of Management & Organization,* 1–20. doi: 10.1017/jmo.2022.95	Leclerc, Kennedy, & Campis (2021)	**New Zealand** -Massey University **Malaysia** -Sunway University **Pakistan** -University of Turbat
15	2023	Millenbach, L., Carey, M. G., DeChance, C., Diaz, L., Graham, P., Moorehead, J., Seller, K., & Zajc, M. (2023). NYONL study explores self-care practices. *Nurse Leader, 21*(4), 438–444.	Leclerc, Strenge-McNabb, Thibodeaux, Campis, & Kennedy (2022)	**United States** -Utica University -University of Rochester -Albany Medical Center -Lincoln Hospital -Cochran School of Nursing
16	2023	Östergård, K., Kuha, S., & Kanste, O. (2023). Health-care leaders' and professionals' experiences and perceptions of compassionate leadership: A mixed-methods systematic review. *Leadership in health services (Bradford, England), ahead-of-print* (ahead-of-print), 49–65. doi: 10.1108/LHS-06-2023-0043	Leclerc, Kennedy, & Campis (2020)	**Finland** -University of Oulu -Finland and Finnish Centre for Evidence-Based Health Care
17	2023	Shokry, W. M., Elshall, S. E., & Darwish, S. S. (2023). Nurses' proactive behavior, relational coordination, and professional identity as predictors of head nurses' relational leadership. *Tanta Scientific Journal, 31*(4) (Suppl 2), 58–75.	Leclerc, Kennedy, & Campis (2021)	**Egypt** -Menoufia University
18	2023	Shin, J. Y., & Jang, E. H. (2023). Influence of person-centered perioperative nursing and patient safety competency on patient safety management activities among operation room nurses: A descriptive study. *Korean Journal of Adult Nursing, 35*(2), 97–106.	Kennedy, Campis, & Leclerc (2020)	**Korea** -Catholic Kwandong University -Incheon Catholic University
19	2024	Romano, C. C. (2024). One voice. *Nurse Leader, 22*(6), 778–780.	Kennedy, Leclerc, & Campis (2022)	**United States**
20	2024	Carlucci, A. M., & Fitzpatrick, J. J. (2024). Emotional intelligence: A nurse manager's relationship to a healthy work environment. *Nursing management, 55*(6), 38–44. doi: 10.1097/nmg.0000000000000136	Leclerc, Kennedy, & Campis (2021)	**United States** -University Hospitals—Cleveland Ohio -Case Western Reserve University
21	2024	Hussein Mohamed, I. I., Aref, S. M., Fahmy, A. M., & Ali El-said, H. (2024). Nurses' perception of ethical climate and its relation to workplace deviance behavior. *Minia Scientific Nursing Journal, 16*(2), 31–39.	Lesandrini, & Leclerc (2024)	**Egypt** -Minia University

	Year	Publication	Work Cited	Country—
22	2024	Kämäräinen, P., Mikkola, L., Nurmeksela, A., Wright, M., & Kvist, T. (2024). Nurse leaders' interpersonal communication competence: A mixed-method systematic review. *Journal of Advanced Nursing, 80*, 4372–4394. doi: 10.1111/jan.16184	Leclerc, Strenge-McNabb, Thibodeaux, Campis, & Kennedy (2022)	**Finland** -University of Eastern Finland -Tampere University
23	2024	Kwame, A., & Petrucka, P. M. (2024). Effective nursing leadership as a catalyst for person-centered care and positive nursing-patient interactions: Evidence from a public Ghanaian hospital. *Discover Health Systems, 3*(50). doi: 10.1007/s44250-024-00095-5	Leclerc, Kennedy, & Campis (2020)	**Canada** -University of Saskatchewan
24	2024	Ma, X., Gan, Xiao'er, & Jiang, T. (2024). Exploring factors contributing to high turnover rate among digital film technicians: A grounded theory approach. *SAGE Open, 14*(4). doi :10.1177/21582440241271227	Leclerc, Kennedy, & Campis (2021)	**China** -South China Normal University
25	2024	McClung, E. L., & Gaberson, K. B. (2024). Confronting punishment of errors with a "Just Culture" environment. *Nursing, 54*(7), 60.	Kennedy, Leclerc, & Campis (2023)	**United States** -University Hospitals—Cleveland, OH -Duquesne University, Pittsburgh, PA
26	2024	Narzikul, T. D., & O'Connor, M. (2024). Systems caring: Guiding principles for leaders. *Nurse Leader, 22*(3), 295–297.	Leclerc, Kennedy, & Campis (2021)	**United States** -Villanova University, Philadelphia, PA
27	2024	Reyes-Walsh, L. M., Lee, M., Dyess, S., Myers, R. E., Beidler, S., Willet, J., Whiddon, A., Garringer, M., & Porter, K. (2024). Harmonizing perspectives: An interdisciplinary approach to developing a multidimensional theoretical framework of self-care for student success. *Journal of Higher Education Theory and Practice, 24*(11), 193–212.	Kennedy, Leclerc, & Campis (2021)	**United States** -Kennesaw State University,Kennesaw, GA
28	2024	Richards-Green, S., Gough, S., & Mickan, S. (2024). Being an wholistic and developmental healthcare leader: Insights from a grounded theory research study. *Asia Pacific Journal of Health Management, 19*(3), i3255. doi:10.24083/apjhm.v19i3.3255	Leclerc, Kennedy, & Campis (2021)	**Australia** -Bond University

	Year	Publication	Work Cited	Country—
29	2024	Wang, H., Wang, Z., Chen, C., & Wei, W. (2024). Cross-cultural adaptation and psychometric evaluation of the Chinese version of the authentic nurse leadership questionnaire. *Journal of Nursing Management,* 1–10. doi: 10.1155/2024/9996979	Leclerc, Strenge-McNabb, Thibodeaux, Campis, & Kennedy (2022)	**China** -Zhengzhou University -Zhengzhou University People's Hospital **United States** -University of Connecticut School of Nursing
30	2024	Wolf, Z. R., Wright, M. E., Grobbel, C., & Hilton, N. (2024). Critical incidents of nimble, caring leaders: A descriptive qualitative study. *International Journal for Human Caring, 28*(2), 98–108.	Leclerc, Kennedy, & Campis (2021)	**United States** -La Salle University -Clemson University -Oakland University -HCA Florida St. Lucie Medical Center
31	2025	Cunningham, T., & Prestia, A. S. (2025). Removing the golden handcuffs: A leader responds to moral injury. *Nurse Leader, 23*(3), 302–304. doi: 10.1016/j.mnl.2024.12.007	Leclerc, Kennedy, & Campis (2021)	**United States** -Emory University -Florida Atlantic University
32	2025	Alnomasy, N., Pangket, P., Alreshidi, B., Alrashidi, H., Shinners, L., Alsaqri, S., & Mostoles, R. J. (2025). Artificial intelligence in healthcare: Assessing impact on professional roles and preparedness among hospital nurse leaders. *Digital Health, 1*(1), 1–15. doi: 10.1177/20552076251356362	Lesandrini, & Leclerc (2024)	**Saudi Arabia** -College of Nursing University of Ha'il -Dept. of Community & Mental Health, Taif University **Australia** -Southern Cross University, Gold Coast Campus
33	2025	Lunn, C., O' Donnell, C., MacCurtain, S., & Coffey, A. (2025). Realigning identity: Nurse executives' experiences within a new socio-professional group - A classic grounded theory study. *International Journal of Nursing Studies Advances, 9,* 100367. doi: 10.1016/j.ijnsa.2025.100367	Leclerc, Kennedy, & Campis (2021)	**Ireland** -University of Limerick (School of Nursing & Midwifery; Kemmy Business School; Heath Research Institute)
34	2025	Williams, K. & Murray, D. (2025, August). Proposing grounded theory as a method to facilitate and extend reflective practice. *Higher Education.* doi: 10.1007/s10734-025-01516-x	Leclerc, Kennedy, & Campis (2021)	**Australia** -University of South Australia, Adelaide
35	2025	Döner, E. & Efeoğlu, E. (2025). A perspective on the concepts of compassion and mercy in the context of adapting the compassionate leadership scale to Turkish culture. *Journal of Social and Economic Research, 27*(49), 685–709.	Leclerc, Kennedy, & Campis (2021)	**Turkey** - Adana, Turkey, Alparslan Türkeş University of Science and Technology, Faculty of Economics, Administrative and Social Sciences, Department of Business Administration

	Year	Publication	Work Cited	Country—
36	2025	Moreno, J.T.M. (2025). Aesthetic leadership in nursing: A theoretical proposal for rehumanizing care delivery. *Nursing Inquiry, 32*(3), e70034. doi: 10.1111/nin .70034	Leclerc, Kennedy, & Campis (2020)	**Spain** -University of the Balearic
37	2025	Kourkouni, V., Galanis, P., Athanasakis, K., & Igoumenidis, M. (2025, June 20). Impact of ethical leadership and organizational culture on nursing personnel's organizational commitment: a cross-sectional study. *Cureus, 17*(6): e86440. doi: 10.7759/cureus.86440	Lesandrini & Leclerc (2024)	**Greece** -University of Patras, Dept. of Nursing -University of Athens, Clinical Epidemiology Lab -University of West Attica, Dept. of Public Health Policy
38	2025	Silva, L.F., Migallos, S.F., Baleña, S. B., & Chavez, F. C. (2025). A structural equation model on nurses' capacity management system. *International Journal of Novel Research and Development, 10*(4). doi: 10.56975/ijnrd.v10i4.305998	Leclerc, Kennedy, & Campis (2021)	**Philippines** San Pedro College
39	2025	Nelson, A., & Serratt, T. (2025). Building belonging: Transforming ICU nurse orientation through relational leadership and shared governance. *Nursing Management*, *56*(7), 18–28. doi: 10.1097 /nmg.0000000000000273	Leclerc, Strenge-McNabb, Thibodeaux, Campis, & Kennedy (2022)	**United States** -University of Oklahoma, College of Nursing
40	2025	Wu, Y., Chen, W., Zhang, R., Yang, Y., Wang, H., Xu, Y., & Zang, S. (2025). The chain mediating roles of professional identity and workplace social capital in the relationship between inclusive leadership and burnout of nurses: A longitudinal study. *Journal of Nursing Management*. Article ID 4713030. doi: 10.1155/jonm /4713030	Leclerc, Strenge-McNabb, Thibodeaux, Campis, & Kennedy (2022)	**China** -China Medical University, Dept. of Community Nursing -Jilin University, SON -Wuhan University, School of Politics & Public Administration -Baoding No. 4 Central Hospital Research & Education Dept. -Shandong University, School of Nursing & Rehab The First Hospital of China Medical University, Dept. of Radiology

APPENDIX C

Human-Centered Leadership in Healthcare: Dimensions and Attributes with Definitions

Self	**Practices to support self**
Well-Being	Approaches life satisfaction through a holistic, subjective, and multidimensional approach while finding balance in the elements of physical, emotional, social, spiritual, intellectual, and financial health.
Self-Care	Maintains a healthy relationship with self, focusing on physical, mental, and spiritual care. The way we treat ourselves.
Self-Compassion	Views life struggles with understanding, kindness, and grace. The way we relate to ourselves.
Self-Aware	Understands the underlying intentions that steer our thoughts, actions, and behaviors. The way we see ourselves.
Mindfulness	Checks in with self in the moment to note and acknowledge feelings and thoughts.
Awakener	**Cultivates our people**
Motivator	Establishes a learning culture that leverages the power of the individual's intrinsic motivation.
Coach	Provides honest feedback addressing strengths and opportunities to improve performance.
Mentor	Advises on professional career path and actions to achieve goals.
Architect	Designs structures and processes so innovation can emerge.
Advocate	Ensures resources are available for best practice and professional growth.

Connector	**Builds our community**
Collaborator	Unifies others around shared mission and vision.
Supporter	Supports, recognizes, and appreciates individual contributions.
Edgewalker	Embraces change by supporting experimentation of ideas to generate innovative solutions.
Engineer	Ensures people are positioned within teams to leverage their individual strengths while enhancing overall team performance.
Authentic Communicator	Builds mutual trust through authentic presence, active listening, and speaking with integrity.
Upholder	**Recognizes humanity in others**
Mindful	Focuses attention, awareness, and energy on the present.
Others-Oriented	Supports with respect, kindness, empathy, and empowerment.
Emotionally Aware	Recognizes how emotions influence behavior, communication, and relationships.
Socially and Organizationally Aware	Recognizes context, unwritten rules, and unspoken words to guide interactions.
Personally Well and Healthy	Prioritizes harmony between work and personal life demands to empower others to do the same.

APPENDIX D

Crosswalk of American Nurses Association Code of Ethics for Nurses (2024) with Supporting Culture Created by Human-Centered Leaders

COE Provision	Provision Description	Human-Centered Leadership Dimension	Associated Culture
Provision 1	The nurse practices with compassion and respect for the inherent dignity, worth, and unique attributes of every person.	Upholder	Culture of Caring
Provision 2	A nurse's primary commitment is to the recipient(s) of nursing care, whether an individual, family, group, community, or population.	Upholder	Culture of Caring
Provision 3	The nurse establishes a trusting relationship and advocates for the rights, health, and safety of recipient(s) of nursing care.	Connector Upholder	Culture of Excellence Culture of Caring
Provision 4	Nurses have authority over nursing practice and are responsible and accountable for their practice consistent with their obligations to promote health, prevent illness, and provide optimal care.	Awakener	Culture of Excellence
Provision 5	The nurse has moral duties to self as a person of inherent dignity and worth, including an expectation of a safe place to work that fosters flourishing, authenticity of self at work, and self-respect through integrity and professional competence.	Self Upholder	Culture of Well-Being Culture of Caring

COE Provision	Provision Description	Human-Centered Leadership Dimension	Associated Culture
Provision 6	Nurses, through individual and collective effort, establish, maintain, and improve the ethical environment of the work setting that affects nursing care and the well-being of nurses.	Self Connector	Culture of Well-Being Culture of Trust
Provision 7	Nurses advance the profession through multiple approaches to knowledge development, professional standards, and the generation of policies for nursing, health, and social concerns.	Awakener	Culture of Excellence
Provision 8	Nurses build collaborative relationships and networks with nurses, other healthcare and nonhealthcare disciplines, and the public to achieve greater ends.	Connector	Culture of Trust
Provision 9	Nurses and their professional organizations work to enact and resource practices, policies, and legislation to promote social justice, eliminate health inequities, and facilitate human flourishing.	Awakener Connector Upholder	Culture of Excellence Culture of Trust Culture of Caring
Provision 10	Nursing, through organizations and associations, participates in the global nursing and health community to promote human and environmental health, well-being, and flourishing.	Self Awakener Connector Upholder	Culture of Well-Being Culture of Excellence Culture of Trust Culture of Caring

Note: For a detailed description of the ANA Code of Ethics for Nurses (2024), visit the website: https://codeofethics.ana.org/home

APPENDIX E

Examples of Human-Centered Leadership in Healthcare Practices Aligned with American Nurses Credentialing Center (2023) Magnet Standards

Magnet Standard and Issue	Human-Centered Leadership in Healthcare (HCL-HC) Practice	Dimension of HCL-HC	Outcome	Implications
Peri-pandemic trials, organizational structure changes, and culture shifts require prioritizing relationships, trust, and identity to support a healthy culture.	Integrating HCL-HC into the Nursing Strategic Plan to drive intentional integration throughout Nursing. Starting with the dimension of Self, leaders learn to lead differently, prioritizing their wellness and that of others, and adopting a relational approach.	Self, Awakener, Connector, and Upholder	A specific workstream, named HCL-HC, created an infrastructure to drive the professional development of leaders and the adoption of a common language and leadership approach, with humanity at the heart of nursing practice.	The culture is shifting to incorporate HCL-HC language and behaviors in all aspects of professional nursing, including quality care, patient safety, professional growth, ownership, and innovative problem-solving.

Magnet Standard and Issue	Human-Centered Leadership in Healthcare (HCL-HC) Practice	Dimension of HCL-HC	Outcome	Implications
In the current Volatile, Uncertain, Complex, and Ambiguous environment in healthcare, organizations recognize the need to prioritize inclusivity and belonging, adopting a people-first approach to achieve market-leading outcomes.	The mindful human-centered leader recognizes the basic human needs of "feeling valued and adding value." "Mattering" and respect spark creativity and innovation, which are essential for solving problems that have never been experienced before.	Self, Connector, and Upholder	A sense of belonging fosters engagement, motivation, and innovation, enhancing problem-solving, especially in uncharted territory.	The team experiences psychological safety, where individuals feel empowered to take smart risks, share ideas, and collaborate across disciplines. This impacts both innovation and resilience.
Structural Empowerment	**HCL-HC Practice**	**Dimension of HCL-HC**	**Outcome**	**Implications**
Nurse leaders' annual goals included board certification because very few were certified.	HCL-HC leaders foster professional development and collaborative teamwork by providing financial support, facilitating certification prep, and promoting a non-zero-sum mindset. The team succeeded together.	Awakener and Connector	100% of the nursing leadership team achieved board certification.	Nurse leaders set an example for board certification in the organization.
The organization was struggling with a fall rate above their stated goals.	The human-centered leader fostered problem-solving at the point of care through professional governance. Empowered interprofessional teams developed their process metrics to measure their contribution toward achieving the goal.	Awakener and Connector	The fall rate began to trend downward over a period of five months and held steady at two to three falls per 1,000 patient days.	The interdisciplinary teams owned their processes and outcomes as they contributed to the overall organizational goal. Contributing to and achieving results led to increased trust, accountability, and teamwork.
Exemplary Professional Practice	**HCL-HC Practice**	**Dimension of HCL-HC**	**Outcome**	**Implications**
Lack of professional identity and role clarity of the professional nurse in the postpandemic environment.	Identity upgrade: The nursing team, led by the hospital practice council guided a postpandemic revision of the Nursing Professional Practice Model using HCL-HC as a guiding theory and appreciative inquiry as the change process.	Self, Awakener, Connector, and Upholder	The nursing team clarified their professional identity through professional development and empowered decision-making by experts at the point of care.	Integration of the HCL-HC dimensions of the Professional Practice Model provided a shared mental model for leaders to connect the dots from their leadership actions to the co-creation of a culture of excellence, trust, and caring.

Exemplary Professional Practice	HCL-HC Practice	Dimension of HCL-HC	Outcome	Implications
The organization aimed to align its Relationship-Based Care model at the bedside with leaders' relational leadership (HCL-HC) to foster a unified culture.	The organization closed the gap between nurse leaders and clinical nurses by connecting the bedside Relationship-Based Care delivery model to a relationship-based leadership model (HCL-HC).	Self, Awakener, Connector, and Upholder	HCL-HC was incorporated into nursing orientation, preceptor development training, research, EBP, and innovation initiatives. It influenced shared governance, transition to practice programs, and mentoring programs.	HCL-HC has been consistently integrated into the nursing leadership culture, providing an evidence-based approach to "the way things are done."
New Knowledge Innovations and Improvements	**HCL-HC Practice**	**Dimension of HCL-HC**	**Outcome**	**Implications**
A direct care nurse who was in an academic graduate nursing leadership program introduced HCL-HC to their Director and Chief Nursing Officer. HCL-HC was implemented via on-site appreciative inquiry and virtual workshops with nursing leaders. The program was evaluated for leader utility and associated outcomes.	The program included structured peer coaching, reflective practice sessions, and leadership development workshops designed to equip nurse managers with tools to foster trust, collaboration, and resilience within their teams. Leaders were trained to model self-awareness, active listening, and inclusive decision-making, reinforcing a culture where nurses felt valued and empowered.	Self, Awakener	The program's impact was evaluated through pre- and postintervention assessments measuring nurse engagement, retention, and patient satisfaction. Results showed reduced turnover, stronger team cohesion, and improved patient experiences. Qualitative feedback further highlighted enhanced psychological safety and professional fulfillment, reinforcing relational leadership's role in sustaining a Magnet-designated environment.	The effectiveness of HCL-HC in driving systemic improvements was identified as a central contributor to a culture shift from traditional to relational.

New Knowledge Innovations and Improvements	HCL-HC Practice	Dimension of HCL-HC	Outcome	Implications
A large urban hospital implemented a HCL-HC-based mentoring program to support new graduate registered nurses (NGRNs) transitioning into practice. Recognizing the challenges of burnout, role uncertainty, and retention, leadership sought to create a structured, relational mentorship model that prioritized psychological safety, emotional intelligence, and professional identity development.	The program comprised four main components: 1- Relational Mentoring—Pairing NGRNs with experienced nurse mentors trained in active listening, empathy, and reflective practice to foster trust and psychological safety. 2- Structured Peer Coaching—Monthly guided reflection sessions where NGRNs and mentors discussed challenges, shared insights, and reinforced self-awareness and resilience. 3- Inclusive Decision-Making—Encouraging NGRNs to voice concerns and contribute to unit-based improvements, reinforcing belonging and engagement. 4- Mindfulness and Emotional Intelligence Training—Providing workshops on stress management, self-regulation, and compassionate communication to enhance confidence and adaptability.	Self, Awakener, Connector, Upholder	Outcomes revealed turnover among NGRNs decreased by 18% within the first year. Postprogram surveys showed a 25% increase in nurses feeling safe to ask questions and seek support. Emotional exhaustion scores (measured via the Maslach Burnout Inventory) declined by 30% among NGRNs. Patient Care—HCAHPS scores reflected a 12% improvement in patient satisfaction related to nurse communication and responsiveness.	HCL-HC fosters innovation by tackling workforce challenges through relational mentorship with NGRNs. Prioritizing psychological safety, emotional intelligence, and peer support boosts retention, reduces burnout, and improves patient care. Embedding these principles in mentoring programs strengthens leadership pipelines, ensuring a sustainable nursing workforce.

Reference: American Nurses Credentialing Center. (2023). *Magnet application manual*. ANCC.

APPENDIX F

Crosswalk of American Nurses Credentialing Center (2024) Pathway Standards with Human-Centered Leadership in Healthcare Dimensions and Attributes

Human-Centered Leadership in Healthcare (HCL-HC) Dimension Self	Pathway Standard	HCL-HC Alignment and Real-World Example
Well-Being	**Standard 3: Safety**	Nurse managers model a holistic approach to individual and collective well-being that prioritizes appropriate rest and meal breaks. The nurse manager's behaviors and way of being create the expectation for direct are nurses (DCNs) to do the same.
Self-Care	**Standard 5: Well-Being**	Nurse managers model a healthy relationship with themselves by prioritizing work schedules grounded in well-being for themselves. The nurse manager's behaviors and way of being create the expectation for DCNs to do the same.
Self-Compassion	**Standard 5: Well-Being**	Organizational leaders harness the power of self-compassion to model the way to acknowledge the life struggles of self and others with understanding, kindness, and grace. For example, the chief nursing officer (CNO) creates a peer financial mentoring program for DCNs. The CNO grew up in a single-parent household and recognizes many team members are experiencing the same financial challenges as they did.

Human-Centered Leadership in Healthcare (HCL-HC) Dimension Self	Pathway Standard	HCL-HC Alignment and Real-World Example
Self-Aware	**Standard 1: Shared Decision-Making**	Organizational leaders model self-awareness as a way for interprofessional team members to honor themselves and their intentions in the process of shared decision-making (SDM). For example, the CNO recognizes how collaborating with the chief medical officer to improve interdisciplinary rounds influences how DCNs learn about interprofessional collaboration and decision-making.
Mindfulness	**Standard 6: Professional Development**	DCNs harness the power of self-reflection to acknowledge strengths and areas for growth. For example, during orientation, the DCN does this through formative evaluation (learning needs assessments) every other week and daily debriefing with their preceptor and self.
HCL-HC Dimension Awakener	**Pathway Standard**	**HCL-HC Alignment and Real-World Example**
Motivator	**Standard 5: Well-Being**	Nurse managers appeal to DCNs' intrinsic motivation to harmonize work and personal well-being by allowing creative scheduling models. For example, the nurse manager enables the unit-based SDM council to propose non-traditional shifts, i.e., two, four, six, or 10 hours, which allows for the DCNs to collaborate with the best interest of the patients (safe staffing) alongside equal ranking with DCN well-being.
Coach	**Standard 2: Leadership**	The nurse leader embraces a coaching mindset to receive peer and DCN feedback within the context of performance evaluation. For example, nurse leaders are expected to take part in 360° peer feedback evaluations.
	Standard 6: Professional Development	Organizational leaders provide transition-to-practice programs for New Graduate Nurses (NGNs) and experienced nurses that integrate coaching as a way to create a culture of feedback. For example, NGNs take part in a year-long residency while experienced nurses take part in specialty fellowships.
Mentor	**Standard 2: Leadership**	Based on individual development plans, nurses at all levels are mentored on professional career path and actions to achieve goals. For example, a nursing director guides the professional development of a nurse manager based on individual goals as they align with organizational priorities and strategy.
Architect	**Standard 3: Safety**	Organizational leaders create a psychologically safe structure for team members to report discriminatory behaviors and receive closed-loop communication on actions taken. This could include a designated role with someone uniquely prepared to receive, address, and communicate issues around discriminatory behavior.

HCL-HC Dimension Awakener	Pathway Standard	HCL-HC Alignment and Real-World Example
Advocate	**Standard 1: Shared Decision-Making**	Organizational leaders advocate on behalf of interprofessional team members to voice ethical concerns using organizational structure and process. For example, leaders ensure all nurses are trained and understand how to submit an ethics consult.
	Standard 3: Safety	Nurse leaders advocate for resources to support DCNs to practice safely and effectively when assigned to an area other than their primary area, i.e., proactive cross-training.
HCL-HC Dimension Connector	**Pathway Standard**	**HCL-HC Alignment and Real-World Example**
Collaborator	**Standard 3: Safety**	Organizational leaders collaborate with stakeholders, i.e., Security and Human Resources to ensure policy and practice are aligned for DCNs to be able to enforce said policies when experiencing verbal or physical abuse from patients and visitors.
	Standard 3: Safety	Organizational leaders work together to create a defined and standardized transition process that's safe and grounded in the shared vision and mission for quality patient care, i.e., collaborative partners may include DCNs, providers, EMS, and care coordination.
Supporter	**Standard 4: Quality**	Leaders support DCNs in reporting nurse-related safety events by promoting a culture of trust and psychological safety; leaders support the implementation of strategies created with input from DCNs to prevent these events from reoccurring.
Edgewalker	**Standard 1: Shared Decision-Making**	Organizational leaders encourage innovation to emerge through SDM councils in efforts to address community health needs. For example, based on the hospital's annual community assessment and findings related to neglect and abuse in teen parents, the Women's Services SDM council collaborates with local high schools to develop parenting classes for teens.
Engineer	**Standard 6: Professional Development**	During orientation, the DCN is an active participant in crafting the plan alongside their leader and educator. For example, the DCN completes bi-weekly formative evaluations (learning needs assessments) and identifies time management as an area for growth. The DCN advocates for support from team members who are proficient at time management.

HCL-HC Dimension Connector	Pathway Standard	HCL-HC Alignment and Real-World Example
Authentic Communicator	**Standard 2: Leadership**	Organizational leaders build mutual trust through consistent and persistent authentic communication about prioritization of a positive practice environment during leadership or organizational changes. For example, the CNO is visible and present at SDM council meetings to support professional practice when the hospital has been acquired by a larger health system.

HCL-HC Dimension Upholder	Pathway Standard	HCL-HC Alignment and Real-World Example
Mindful	**Standard 2: Leadership**	The nurse manager harnesses the power of mindfulness, focusing attention and awareness while in the presence of DCNs. For example, the nurse manager sets aside time to round on the unit regularly with the intention of talking with DCNs 1:1 in their clinical environment.
Others-Oriented	**Standard 3: Safety**	Nurse leaders create a structure/environment of empowerment that honors the voice and actions of DCNs in communicating concerns about the long-term nurse staffing plan within the framework of well-being for patients and nurses. For example, the CNO encourages open dialogue within designated "office hours" for 1:1 conversation, town halls, and rounding.
Emotionally Aware	**Standard 4: Quality**	Organizational leaders honor unique customs and practices by bringing awareness to how individual team members' emotions influence behavior, communication, and relationships. This may occur through inclusive leadership practices such as honoring team members' accommodations for religious practices. The leader uses emotional awareness to navigate individual and team responses.
Socially and Organizationally Aware	**Standard 5: Well-Being**	Organizational leaders honor social and organizational rules/guidelines/policies to provide real-time support to staff who've experienced a work-related adverse situation. For example, the CNO recognizes that the ED staff may also be affected by the death of a pediatric patient admitted to the pediatric intensive care unit. The CNO ensures all team members receive appropriate real-time support, i.e., debriefing, Code Lavender.
Personally Well and Healthy	**Standard 1: Shared Decision-Making**	Nurse leaders mentor DCNs in prioritizing personal wellness and health; this empowers DCNs to make well-being a priority for themselves and others. For example, a unit-based SDM council works with the nurse manager to create a program for "wellness mentors" between newly graduated RNs and experienced nurses.

References: (1) Leclerc, L., & Pabico, C. (2023). A blueprint for well-being: Modeling the way through Human-Centered Leadership and Pathway to Excellence. *Nursing Management, 54*(4), 9–16. (2) American Nurses Credentialing Center. (2024). *Pathway to Excellence standards and elements of performance.* ANCC.

APPENDIX G

Crosswalk of American Association of Colleges of Nursing (2021)

The Essentials: Core Competencies for Professional Nursing Education with Human-Centered Leadership in Healthcare Dimensions, Attributes, and Outcomes

DOMAIN 10: PERSONAL, PROFESSIONAL, AND LEADERSHIP DEVELOPMENT

Descriptor: Participation in activities and self-reflection that foster personal health, resilience, and well-being contribute to lifelong learning and support the acquisition of nursing expertise and the assertion of leadership.

Contextual Statement: Competency in personal, professional, and leadership development encompasses three areas: (1) development of the nurse as an individual who is resilient, agile, and capable of adapting to ambiguity and change; (2) development of the nurse as a professional responsible for lifelong learning and ongoing self-reflection; and (3) development of the nurse as a leader proficient in asserting control, influence, and power in professional and personal contexts, which includes advocacy for patients and the nursing profession as leaders within the healthcare arena. Development of these dimensions requires a commitment to personal growth, sustained expansion of professional knowledge and expertise, and determined leadership practice in a variety of contexts. Graduates must develop attributes and skills critical to the viability of the profession and practice environments. The aim is to promote diversity and retention in the profession, self-awareness, avoidance of stress-induced emotional and mental exhaustion, and re-direction of energy from negative perceptions to positive influence through leadership opportunities.

Competencies:

10.1 Demonstrate a commitment to personal health and well-being.

10.2 Demonstrate a spirit of inquiry that fosters flexibility and professional maturity.

10.3 Develop capacity for leadership.

	Description	Human-Centered Leadership: Book Chapter	Dimension	Attribute	Outcome
10.1	Demonstrate a commitment to personal health and well-being.	**Chapter 3**: The Importance of Knowing Our "Why" **Chapter 4**: The Mindset—"It Starts with Me" **Chapter 5**: The Language—"I Matter" **Chapter 9**: The Upholder **Chapter 15**: Positive Practice Environments	Self Upholder	All attributes Personally Well and Healthy, Mindful	Culture of Well-Being Culture of Caring
10.2	Demonstrate a spirit of inquiry that fosters flexibility and professional maturity.	**Chapter 1**: On the Shoulders of Giants **Chapter 2**: Proof in Practice **Chapter 7**: The Awakener **Chapter 11**: Cultural Intelligence **Chapter 12**: Affirmative Disruption **Chapter 13**: Using Systems Thinking to Build Human-Centered Solutions **Chapter 14**: The Architecture of Inclusion **Chapter 18**: Dealing with Joy Interrupters	Awakener	Motivator Coach Mentor Architect Advocate	Culture of Excellence

	Description	Human-Centered Leadership: Book Chapter	Dimension	Attribute	Outcome
10.3	Develop capacity for leadership.	**Chapter 4**: The Mindset—"It Starts with Me" **Chapter 5**: The Language—"I Matter" **Chapter 6**: But It's Not About You! **Chapter 7**: The Awakener **Chapter 8**: The Connector **Chapter 9**: The Upholder **Chapter 15**: Positive Practice Environments	Self Awakener Connector Upholder	Well-Being, Self-Care, Self-Compassion, Self-Aware, Mindfulness Motivator, Coach, Mentor, Advocate, Architect Supporter, Collaborator, Edgewalker, Engineer, Authentic Communicator Personally Well and Healthy, Emotional Awareness, Others-Oriented, Social and Organizational Awareness, Mindful	Culture of Well-Being Culture of Excellence Culture of Trust Culture of Caring Culture of Well-Being, Excellence, Trust, and Caring

Note: For more detailed information on the American Association of Colleges of Nursing (2021) *The Essentials: Core Competencies for Professional Nursing Education*, visit the AACN website: https://www.aacnnursing.org/essentials

APPENDIX H

Crosswalk of the American Association of Critical Care Nurses (2021) Healthy Work Environment Assessment Tool (HWEAT-Team) with Human-Centered Leadership in Healthcare Dimensions, Attributes, and Cultures

HWE Standard	HWEAT—Team Questions Rating scale: Poor—Fair—Good—Very Good—Excellent—Outstanding	Human-Centered Leadership (HCL) Dimension	HCL Culture
Skilled Communication	In my organization, the communication taking place between RNs and top-level leadership (e.g., CNO, CEO, executives, directors) is . . .	**Awakener** (Architect) **Connector** (Authentic Communicator, Collaborator, Supporter, Engineer) **Upholder** (Others-Oriented, Socially/Organizationally Aware)	Excellence Trust Caring
	In my work unit, the communication taking place between RNs and nurse managers is . . .	**Self** (Mindfulness, Self-Aware) **Awakener** (Motivator) **Connector** (Authentic Communicator) **Upholder** (Mindful, Emotionally Aware, Socially/Organizationally Aware)	Well-Being Excellence Trust Caring

HWE Standard	HWEAT—Team Questions Rating scale: Poor—Fair—Good—Very Good—Excellent—Outstanding	Human-Centered Leadership (HCL) Dimension	HCL Culture
	In my work unit, the communication taking place between RNs and other healthcare colleagues (e.g., other RNs, physicians, respiratory therapists, pharmacists, nutrition services, social workers, physical therapists, etc.) is . . .	**Connector** (Authentic Communicator, Collaborator) **Upholder** (Mindful, Others-Oriented, Socially/Organizationally Aware)	Trust Caring
	In my work unit, RNs make sure their actions match their words.	**Self** (Self-Awareness) **Connector** (Authentic Communicator) **Upholder** (Mindful)	Well-Being Trust Caring
True Collaboration	In my organization, the collaboration taking place between RNs and top-level leadership (e.g., CNO, CEO, executives, directors) is . . .	**Awakener** (Advocate) **Connector** (Collaborator, Authentic Communicator) **Upholder** (Socially/Organizationally Aware)	Excellence Trust Caring
	In my work unit, the collaboration taking place between RNs and nurse managers is . . .	**Connector** (Collaborator, Authentic Communicator)	Trust
	In my work unit, the collaboration taking place between RNs and other healthcare colleagues (e.g., other RNs, physicians, respiratory therapists, pharmacists, nutrition services, social workers, physical therapists, etc.) is . . .	**Connector** (Collaborator, Engineer)	Trust
	In my work unit, when disputes among healthcare team members occur, there are processes in place that help resolve them.	**Connector** (Authentic Communicator, Engineer)	Trust
Effective Decision-Making	In my organization, RNs influence organization-level decisions that affect the quality of patient care.	**Awakener** (Architect, Advocate) **Connector** (Supporter, Engineer)	Excellence Trust

HWE Standard	HWEAT—Team Questions Rating scale: Poor—Fair—Good—Very Good—Excellent—Outstanding	Human-Centered Leadership (HCL) Dimension	HCL Culture
	In my work unit, RNs and other healthcare team members are involved in making patient care decisions.	**Connector** (Collaborator, Engineer, Authentic Communicator) **Upholder** (Others-Oriented, Socially/Organizationally Aware)	Trust Caring
	In my work unit, patients and their families are provided the opportunity to participate in decisions affecting their care.	**Connector** (Collaborator) **Upholder** (Others-Oriented, Emotionally Aware)	Trust Caring
	In my work unit, RNs are valued partners in influencing unit processes.	**Awakener** (Advocate) **Connector** (Collaborator, Engineer, Supporter)	Excellence Trust
Appropriate Staffing	In my organization, there are staffing policies in place that help support RNs in providing high-quality care.	**Awakener** (Advocate) **Connector** (Collaborator)	Excellence Trust
	In my work unit, there is adequate support staff in place to allow RNs to focus on nursing care.	**Awakener** **Connector** (Collaborator) **Upholder** (Socially/Organizationally Aware)	Excellence Trust Caring
	In my work unit, processes are in place to evaluate the impact of staffing decisions.	**Awakener** (Architect) **Connector** (Engineer)	Excellence Trust
	In my work unit, RN staffing ensures alignment between patient needs and nurse competencies.	**Awakener** (Advocate, Architect) **Connector** (Engineer, Supporter) **Upholder** (Others-Oriented, Mindful, Socially/Organizationally Aware)	Excellence Trust Caring
Meaningful Recognition	In my organization, the recognition taking place between RNs and top-level leadership (e.g., CNO, CEO, executives, directors) is . . .	**Connector** (Advocate) **Upholder** (Others-Oriented, Socially/Organizationally Aware)	Trust Caring
	In my work unit, the recognition taking place between RNs and nurse managers is . . .	**Self** (Mindful) **Awakener** (Advocate) **Connector** (Supporter) **Upholder** (Others-Oriented, Socially/Organizationally Aware)	Excellence Trust Caring

HWE Standard	HWEAT—Team Questions Rating scale: Poor—Fair—Good—Very Good—Excellent—Outstanding	Human-Centered Leadership (HCL) Dimension	HCL Culture
	In my work unit, RNs recognize other healthcare colleagues for their valuable contributions.	**Self** (Self-Awareness) **Awakener** (Motivator, Advocate) **Connector** (Collaborator, Supporter, Authentic Communicator) **Upholder** (Mindful, Others-Oriented, Socially/Organizationally Aware)	Excellence Trust Caring
	In my work unit, other healthcare colleagues recognize RNs for their valuable contributions.	**Self** (Self-Awareness) **Connector** (Supporter, Collaborator) **Upholder** (Mindful, Socially/Organizationally Aware)	Trust Caring
Authentic Leadership	In my organization, the promotion of a professional practice environment by top-level leadership (e.g., CNO, CEO, executives, directors) is . . .	**Awakener** (Motivator, Architect, Advocate) **Connector** (Collaborator, Supporter, Engineer) **Upholder** (Socially/Organizationally Aware, Personally Well and Healthy)	Excellence Trust Caring
	In my work unit, the team members accountable for leading us inspire others to help achieve a healthy work environment.	**Self** (Self-Compassion, Self-Awareness, Mindfulness) **Awakener** (Motivator, Coach, Mentor, Architect, Advocate) **Connector** (Collaborator, Supporter, Edgewalker, Engineer) **Upholder** (Others-Oriented, Personally Well and Healthy)	Well-Being Excellence Trust Caring
	In my work unit, the team members accountable for leading us ensure staff have what they need to do their job.	**Awakener** (Advocate, Architect) **Connector** (Collaborator, Supporter, Engineer) **Upholder** (Others-Oriented)	Excellence Trust Caring
	In my work unit, the team members accountable for leading us effectively address abusive behavior.	**Self** (Mindfulness, Self-Care, Self-Compassion, Self-Awareness, Well-Being) **Awakener** (Advocate) **Connector** (Supporter, Authentic Communicator) **Upholder** (Mindful, Others-Oriented, Emotionally Aware, Socially/Organizationally Aware, Personally Well and Healthy)	Well-Being Excellence Trust Caring

Note: For more detailed information on the AACN. (2021). *AACN standards for establishing and sustaining healthy work environments: Journey to excellence* (2nd ed.), please visit the AACN website: https://www.aacn.org/nursing-excellence/healthy-work-environments

APPENDIX I

Crosswalk of the American Organization of Nurse Leaders (2022) Competencies with Human-Centered Leadership in Healthcare Essentials Leadership Program

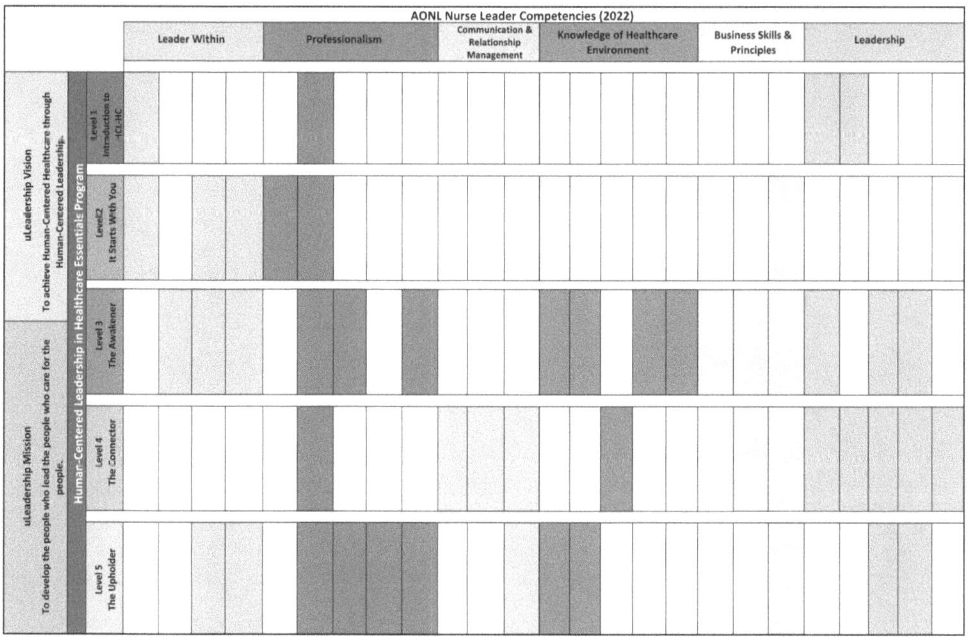

Reference: American Organization of Nurse Leaders (AONL). (2022). AONL Nurse Leader Core Competencies. AONL. Accessed from www.aonl.org/competencies

APPENDIX J

Crosswalk of Relational Leadership Styles and Human-Centered Leadership in Healthcare Dimensions and Attributes

This crosswalk explores the alignment between Human-Centered Leadership in Healthcare (HCL-HC) and the three borrowed leadership styles historically used in healthcare. HCL-HC integrates ideas from all three styles, bringing together a comprehensive way of leading specific to complex healthcare environments. The crosswalk demonstrates how HCL-HC is inclusive of the other relational leadership styles while being unique with attributes specific to healthcare. Of note, is the lack of alignment between transformational leadership and the dimension of Self.

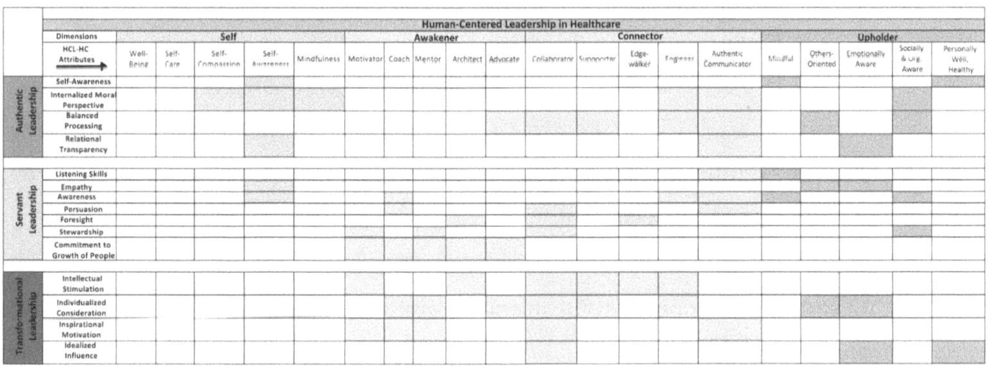

		Human-Centered Leadership in Healthcare																			
	Dimensions	Self					Awakener					Connector					Upholder				
	HCL-HC Attributes →	Well-Being	Self-Care	Self-Compassion	Self-Awareness	Mindfulness	Motivator	Coach	Mentor	Architect	Advocate	Collaborator	Supporter	Edge-walker	Engineer	Authentic Communicator	Mindful	Others-Oriented	Emotionally Aware	Socially & Org. Aware	Personally Well, Healthy
Authentic Leadership	Self-Awareness																				
	Internalized Moral Perspective																				
	Balanced Processing																				
	Relational Transparency																				
Servant Leadership	Listening Skills																				
	Empathy																				
	Awareness																				
	Persuasion																				
	Foresight																				
	Stewardship																				
	Commitment to Growth of People																				
Transformational Leadership	Intellectual Stimulation																				
	Individualized Consideration																				
	Inspirational Motivation																				
	Idealized Influence																				

Note: Fitzpatrick, J., Raso, R., Bailey, K. D., Kennedy, K., & Leclerc, L. (2024, April). *Should nursing abandon transformational leadership: Moving toward a new relational leadership paradigm.* Podium Presentation at the AONL 2024 Inspiring Leaders Conference in New Orleans, LA.

LITERATURE SUPPORTING RELATIONAL CROSSWALK

Authentic Leadership

Avolio, B. J., Gardner, W. L., Walumbwa, F. O., Luthans, F., & May, D. R. (2004). Unlocking the mask: A look at the process by which authentic leaders impact follower attitudes and behaviors. *The Leadership Quarterly, 15*(6), 801–823.

Bailey, K. D. (2019). *Examination of authentic leadership in nurse executives in Magnet and non-Magnet hospitals: A correlational study University of Phoenix.* ProQuest Dissertations Publishing, 275452020.

Giordano-Mulligan, M., & Eckardt, S. (2019). Authentic nurse leadership conceptual framework: Nurses' perception of authentic nurse leader attributes. *Nursing Administration Quarterly, 43*(2), 164–174. doi: 10.1097/NAQ.0000000000000344

Northouse, P. G. (2019). *Leadership* (8th ed.). Sage.

Raso, R., Fitzpatrick, J. J., & Masick, K. (2020). Clinical nurses' perceptions of authentic nurse leadership and healthy work environment. *JONA: The Journal of Nursing Administration, 50*(9), 489–494. doi: 10.1097/NNA.0000000000000921

Raso, R., Fitzpatrick, J. J., Masick, K., Giordano-Mulligan, M., & Sweeney, C. D. (2021). Perceptions of authentic nurse leadership and work environment and the pandemic impact for nurse leaders and clinical nurses. *JONA: The Journal of Nursing Administration, 51*(5), 257–263. doi: 10.1097/nna.0000000000001010

Servant Leadership

Greenleaf, R. K. (1977). *Servant leadership: A journey into the nature of legitimate power and greatness.* Paulist Press.

Hall, H. H. (2015). *An exploration of the relationship between servant leadership characteristics of nurse leaders and the perception of empowerment among their followers.* [Doctoral dissertation, Indiana Wesleyan University] ProQuest Networked Digital Library of Theses & Dissertations.

Liao, C., Lee, H. W., Johnson, R. E., & Lin, S. H. (J.) (2020). Serving you depletes me? A leader-centric examination of servant leadership behaviors. *Journal of Management.* doi: 10.1177/0149206320906883

O'Brien, M. E. (2011). *Servant leadership in nursing: Spirituality and practice in contemporary health care.* Jones & Bartlett.

Parris, D. L., & Peachey, J. W. (2013). A systematic literature review of servant leadership theory in organizational contexts. *Journal of Business Ethics, 113*, 377–393.

Transformational Leadership

Bass, B. M. (1985). *Leadership and performance beyond expectations.* Free Press.

Burns, J. M. (1978). *Leadership* (1st ed.). Harper & Row.

Fischer, S. (2016). Transformational leadership in nursing: A concept analysis. *Journal of Advanced Nursing, 72*(11), 2644–2653.

Lanaj, K., Johnson, R. E., & Lee, S. M. (2016). Benefits of transformational behaviors for leaders: A daily investigation of leader behaviors and need fulfillment. *Journal of Applied Psychology, 101*, 237–251.

Lin, S., Scott, B. A., & Matta, F. K. (2019). The dark side of transformational leader behaviors for leaders themselves: A conservation of resources perspective. *Academy of Management Journal, 62*(5), 1556–1582. doi: 10.5465/amj.2016.1255

APPENDIX K

Crosswalk of Watson's Caring Science Caritas (2018) with Human-Centered Leadership in Healthcare Dimensions and Attributes

Human-Centered Leadership in Healthcare			Caritas Process 1	Caritas Process 2	Caritas Process 3	Caritas Process 4	Caritas Process 5	Caritas Process 6	Caritas Process 7	Caritas Process 8	Caritas Process 9	Caritas Process 10
			Sustaining humanistic-altruistic values by practice of loving kindness, compassion and equanimity with self and others.	Being Authentically present, enabling faith/hope/belief system; honoring subjective inner, life-world of self/others.	Being sensitive to self and others by cultivating own spiritual practices; beyond ego-self to transpersonal presence.	Developing and sustaining loving, trusting-caring relationships.	Allowing for expression of positive and negative feelings-authentically listening to another person's story	Creatively problem-solving, 'solution-seeking' through caring process; full use of self and artistry of caring-healing practices via use of all ways of knowing/being/doing/becoming	Engaging in transpersonal teaching and learning within context of caring relationship; staying within others frame of reference-shift toward coaching model for expanded health/wellness	Creating a healing environment at all levels; subtle environment for energetic authentic caring presence.	Reverentially assisting with basic needs as sacred acts, touching mind, body, spirit of others; sustaining human dignity	Opening to spiritual, mystery, unknowns-allowing for miracles
		Practices to Support Self										
Dimension One SELF "I Matter"	Sense of Well-Being	Approaches life satisfaction through a holistic, subjective, and multidimensional approach while finding balance in the elements of physical, emotional, social, spiritual, intellectual, and financial health.										
	Self-Aware	Understands the underlying intentions that steer our thoughts, actions, and behaviors. The way we see ourselves.										
	Self-Compassionate	Views life struggles with understanding, kindness, and grace. The way we relate to ourselves.										
	Self-Nurturing	Maintains a healthy relationship with self, focusing on physical, mental, and spiritual care. The way we treat ourselves.										
	Mindfulness	Checks in with self in the moment to note and acknowledge feelings and thoughts.										
		Cultivates the People										
Dimension Two AWAKENER "I Believe in You"	Motivator	Establishes a learning culture that leverages the power of the individual's intrinsic motivation.										
	Coach	Provides honest feedback addressing strengths and opportunities to improve performance.										
	Mentor	Advises on professional career path and actions to achieve goals.										
	Architect	Designs structures and processes so innovation can emerge.										
	Advocate	Ensures resources are available for best practice and professional growth.										
		Builds the Community										
Dimension Three CONNECTOR "I Trust You"	Collaborator	Unifies others around shared mission and vision.										
	Supporter	Supports, recognizes, and appreciates individual contributions.										
	Edgewalker	Embraces change by supporting experimentation of ideas to generate innovative solutions.										
	Engineer	Ensures people are positioned within teams to leverage their individual strengths while enhancing overall team performance.										
	Authentic Communicator	Builds mutual trust through authentic presence, active listening, and speaking with integrity.										
		Recognizes Humanity in Self and Others										
Dimension Four UPHOLDER "I See You"	Mindful	Focuses attention, awareness, and energy on the present										
	Others-Oriented	Supports with respect, kindness, empathy, and empowerment.										
	Emotionally Aware	Recognizes how emotions influence behavior, communication, and relationships.										
	Socially & Organizationally Aware	Recognizes context, unwritten rules, and unspoken words to guide interactions.										
	Personally Well and Healthy	Prioritizes harmony between work and personal life demands to empower others to do the same.										

REFERENCE

Sitzman, K., & Watson, J. (2018). *Caring Science, Mindful Practice: Implementing Watson's Human Caring Theory* (2nd ed.). Springer.

About the Authors

Lucy Leclerc is a nurse executive, entrepreneur, and chief innovation officer at uLeadership, LLC. She is also a nurse scientist at Emory Healthcare, where she mentors and coaches direct care nurses and interprofessional teams on research, innovation, and evidence-based practice. Her program of research focuses on nursing leadership in practice and academia with an aim to explore the connection between leadership behaviors and outcomes. She is adjunct faculty at the Emory Nell Hodgson Woodruff School of Nursing at Emory University and the Frances Payne Bolton School of Nursing at Case Western Reserve University. She also serves on the editorial board of the *Journal of Nursing Education* and provides peer review for multiple other professional journals. Lucy's "why" in her body of work and in everyday nursing leadership is to reveal what already exists within nurses and nursing teams . . . excellence and professionalism.

Kay Kennedy is a nurse executive, educator, and entrepreneur. By combining a love for nurses, patients, and quality improvement, she has led large nursing teams to create healthy work environments, satisfied patients, and consistent, high-quality care. With experience ranging from bedside nursing to chief nursing officer, she also serves as adjunct faculty at the Nell Hodgson Woodruff School of Nursing at Emory University, MGH Institute of Health Professions, and the Frances Payne Bolton School of Nursing at Case Western Reserve University. She is the CEO of uLeadership, LLC, an internationally recognized professional development and research organization. Her passion as a leader is to ignite innovative problem-solving, develop others to be their best, and lead with empathy and service.

Susan Campis, MSN, RN, NE-BC, NBC-HWC, is a nurse leader, author, health and wellness coach, and serves as chief wellness officer for uLeadership, LLC. Throughout her leadership journey, she has developed a strong passion for coaching and mentoring, helping nursing teams thrive in their roles while delivering outstanding care to patients and their families. As a health and wellness coach, she recognizes that personal well-being is the foundation of professional and personal success. She is committed to fostering a culture of excellence, trust, and caring. Her passion as a leader is to co-create and sustain an environment where every team member has the opportunity to flourish and thrive.

FSC
www.fsc.org
MIX
Papier | Fördert gute Waldnutzung
FSC® C083411

Zeitfracht Medien GmbH
Ferdinand-Jühlke-Straße 7
99095 Erfurt, Deutschland
produktsicherheit@kolibri360.de